To Rich Henderson —
May God be with
you —

Danny Hunbaby

YEA THOUGH I WALK

Published by

Darrell and Lisa Huckaby

2755 Ebenezer Rd

Conyers, GA 30094

Darrell Huckaby

Yea Though I Walk

Copyright 2012

Printed in the United States of America

First Edition

ISBN 978-1-4675-4662-1

YEA THOUGH I WALK

Darrell Huckaby

Author's Note

This book is not a medical journal and I am not attempting to offer medical advice to anyone. Every case of cancer is different and every cancer victim should seek the very best medical advice he or she can find. In the pages of this book I have told my story—as openly and honestly as I know how. I pray that it will bring hope to others. I hope that it will make people laugh and think.

I offer my undying gratitude to all the people who have helped to make this book possible, especially my children, Jamie, Jackson and Jenna—and, of course, my lovely wife Lisa, who did the lay-out for me. The folks at The Adsmith, in Athens, have been unbelievably easy to work with, as always, and my love, admiration and thanks goes out to Aimee Aldrich Jones, my editor.

More than anything else, I hope it will glorify God and reveal to those who may not know—and remind those who already do—of the incredible power of prayer.

Darrell Huckaby

Dedicated to

The Glory of God,

and to all the prayer warriors

who have loved me through this ordeal.

Psalms 23

The LORD is my shepherd; I shall not want.

*He maketh me to lie down in green pastures:
he leadeth me beside the still waters.*

*He restoreth my soul: he leadeth me in the
paths of righteousness for his name's sake.*

*Yea, though I walk through the valley of
the shadow of death, I will fear no evil:
for thou art with me; thy rod and
thy staff they comfort me.*

*Thou preparest a table before me
in the presence of mine enemies:
thou anointest my head with oil;
my cup runneth over.*

*Surely goodness and mercy shall follow me
all the days of my life: and I will dwell
in the house of the LORD forever.*

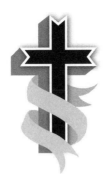

PROLOGUE

You hear those dreaded words, "I'm afraid you have cancer," and a thousand questions pop into your head and a thousand thoughts cross your mind and a thousand emotions flood your soul. If you are like me, not many of the thoughts, questions, or emotions are of a positive nature.

I was sitting in the pre-admission department of our local hospital, preparing for a totally unrelated surgery, when I heard those words. My doctor called me on my cell phone to let me know that we had bigger fish to fry than the gall bladder surgery that necessitated my presence at the hospital that day.

Cancer. We all know someone—or many someones—who has fought and defeated that dastardly disease. We all know others who have fought just as valiantly as our survivor friends and still succumbed. Cancer is no respecter of age or station in life. It is an equal opportunity killer that attacks the young and old, the rich and poor, the weak and the strong. There is no color or creed or ethnic background that can render one safe from cancer.

When I was diagnosed, I wanted information. I wanted to know as much as I could about the disease I was about to fight. I wanted to know the strengths and the weaknesses of my opponent. I wanted to know who my greatest allies were. I wanted to give myself the very best chance at survival because I really enjoy life and want to experience as much of it on this earth as I can. I tried to find people to talk to, people who had experienced what I was about to experience. I wanted to know what to expect.

I found a lot of wonderful, helpful people who were willing to share their experiences with me, but I also learned that no two cancer cases are exactly alike. I pored through the Internet looking for hope and reassurance. I tried the best I could to educate myself. I wanted to know everything there was to know about prostate cancer.

I found site after site after site that gave me all sorts of medical statistics, mostly written in jargon that was very difficult for me to understand. I could read the numbers and compare them to mine and knew enough to know that I didn't usually like what I had read. I found out more than I could comprehend about the medical treatments available to fight prostate cancer, along with the holistic treatments and diets that some people swore by and others discounted. I even found out that if I ate a lemon every day, cancer couldn't touch me. I discounted that theory because I have eaten a lemon every day for the past fifty years.

What I couldn't find was a book that was readable and entertaining and easy to understand, written by someone who had experienced the same emotions I had, someone who had asked the same questions I asked, and thought the same thoughts—someone who could give me a glimpse into the world I was about to enter. I promised myself and my wife and the Lord that if I survived long enough, I would write such a book—a book that would bring hope and information and reassurance, and perhaps a laugh or two, to people who had heard their own doctors proclaim, "I am afraid you have cancer."

This is that book. It is not a medical journal in any way, shape, or form. Nor is it intended as a recommendation for what course someone else might take in dealing with his or her own disease. It is just one man's story—my own. And since I enjoy telling stories and reminiscing, I will certainly take you on more than a few detours as I retrace the steps of my journey.

I hope you enjoy, I hope you relate, I hope you gain a bit of insight into your own situation but, most of all, I hope that I help give you hope. When hope is gone there is nothing else.

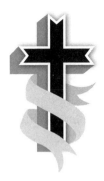

CHAPTER ONE

This isn't the book I intended to write. When I was diagnosed with prostate cancer in late spring of 2011, I wasn't particularly concerned. I had heard all the glib comments everyone has heard about prostate cancer. In my ignorance, I had probably uttered most of them myself.

"If you are going to have cancer, prostate cancer is the best kind to have."

"Prostate cancer advances so slowly that more men die with prostate cancer than from it."

"It's not a matter of if but when a man is going to get prostate cancer."

And my personal favorite, from a good friend: "Piece of cake."

Here are some things I learned. There is no good kind of cancer. Many men die of prostate cancer—about 28,000 a year in the United States alone. It is the second most deadly type of cancer for men, behind lung cancer. Let me assure you, if what I have gone through so far is a piece of cake, I don't want to have dessert at my friend's house any time soon. And lastly, if I have learned anything during my ongoing battle with prostate cancer, it is that nothing ever seems to go as planned.

But back to the book I had intended to write. When I was first diagnosed and before I realized that my male organs were trying to kill me, I thought I would write a little light-hearted paperback about my experiences. I thought it would make folks laugh a little and help men—and their families—who were facing the same thing I was facing understand what they were about to experience.

Always one to get the cart before the horse, I even began to visualize the cover. It would feature a photograph of yours truly, grinning like a mule eating briers, wearing a blue hospital gown and holding on to one of those moving IV poles. I even sent my friend Kathy Hope in search of just the right color gown. The title of the book would be You Took Out My What?!?

As days turned into weeks and weeks into months and then we moved into the second year of the fight, I realized that there would be no easy solution to my problem. As I found myself in a life or death struggle with the dreaded disease that originally I viewed so casually, I realized that there was nothing light-hearted about the war cancer was waging inside my body. Time after time after time my various doctors began conversations with, "I'm sorry but it looks like . . ."

You really never want to have your doctor begin a conversation about your condition with, "I'm sorry but it looks like . . ."

As the days drew on and various procedures and treatments failed to work, my confidence turned to anxiety, then to fear and depression, and finally to despondency and desperation. As Abraham Lincoln once noted, "I was driven to my knees when I had nowhere else to go." I began, more and more, to put my hope where my hope should have been all along—squarely at the foot of the cross. I turned to God when I had nowhere else to turn and soon found myself on a remarkable journey that would lead me on a clear path toward that perfect peace that passes all understanding.

During the darkest days of my ordeal I became so racked with pain and so devoid of energy that I was sometimes convinced each day would be my last. Some days I wished the previous day had been. I would lie in bed at night searching for the right prayer to pray. Tears would flow and I would fall asleep counting not my blessings, but the things on my bucket list—watching my children get married, playing with my grandchildren, celebrating a Bowl Championship Series victory with my beloved Georgia Bulldogs—that I thought I would never live to experience. Often I could not even find the words with which to petition God for comfort and healing. During those bad times I would simply recite scriptures that I had learned as a small boy.

"Our Father who art in heaven, hallowed be thy name . . ."

"I will lift up mine eyes unto the hills."

And every night—and many times during the day—I would find comfort in the words of the shepherd boy who would become king, "The Lord is my shepherd, I shall not want."

The Twenty-third Psalm became my touchstone. If we are honest with ourselves and one another, everyone who has been diagnosed with any kind of cancer begins to think about death. As I began to feel worse and worse, I thought about the possibility of death more and more frequently and those words of David brought more and more comfort to me.

"Yea, though I walk through the valley of the shadow of death, I will fear no evil."

Eventually, I made such a strong connection with my Creator that I came to realize something that I had actually known since I first accepted Christ as a young boy in the Methodist church at Porterdale. I had nothing to fear from life or death as long as I was in a right relation with the Almighty and was living in God's will.

I didn't know if I could beat cancer, but I knew it wouldn't matter if I did or didn't if I were not right with God. And I knew that I could get right with God.

This is the story of my battle with cancer and I hope that it will, indeed, make folks laugh a little and help those who are facing the same thing I was—and my family was—better understand what they might be about to experience. I also hope it will provide a laugh or two, because laughter really is pretty good medicine.

And I hope that it will glorify God because it is only by the grace of God and God's willingness to give an affirming answer to the thousands of prayers that have gone up and continue to go up on my behalf, that I am still around and able to put my story on paper.

Yea Though I Walk. It really is quite a journey. I hope you'll enjoy reliving it with me.

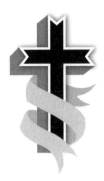

CHAPTER TWO

My buddy Gary says it all started when I fell off the ladder in October of 2010. Let me tell you about that.

We had an ugly old pine tree in our front yard that my lovely wife Lisa wanted cut down. She said it was keeping the grass from growing in our front yard. Understand, we have a yard not a lawn. Have you ever seen before-and-after ads for lawn chemicals? The before picture has crabgrass and dandelions and every weed known to man. The after picture is a manicured lawn that would make the head groundskeeper at Augusta National proud.

Our yard is the before picture. Pine tree or no pine tree, our yard wasn't going to look like the after shot. But since Lisa controls 85 percent of the money and 100 percent of the sex in my life, what Lisa wants, Lisa gets.

That is why I was standing on the top rung of an eight-foot ladder on a splendid October afternoon with a chain saw in my hands. I know. I know. I never have claimed to be the brightest bulb in the chandelier. But before we could cut down the tree—"we" being my father-in-law, Benny, and my brother-in-law, Eddie—I needed to trim some of the larger branches. It seemed like a good idea at the time.

Well, I trimmed the branch. I did indeed. And when it let loose of the tree, the branch came right toward my face. Thankfully I had the presence of mind to throw the chain saw in the opposite direction of where I was going to fall, just about a split second before the branch I had severed hit me square in the face. I landed flat on my back and my head hit the ground—hard.

When I came to, Lisa was standing over me with a mirror so I could decide for myself if I looked as stupid as I apparently was. I was able to stand up and, thankfully nothing was broken. We went to the doctor's office and got checked out and then we went to the hospital for a series of tests. They examined my brain and didn't find anything. Yeah, I know. I think it was Dizzy Dean's brother Paul who used that line first, right after Ol' Diz had been beaned by a fastball. Nothing was broken and that was that—or so I thought.

A couple of weeks after my self-inflicted tumble from the ladder, I started having severe pains in my abdomen and chest wall. It was a strange sensation and very hard to pinpoint. Sometimes it was a dull ache and at other times there were sharp shooting pains. Sometimes I felt extremely bloated and at other times I did not, but the pain was always there. It wasn't excruciating or debilitating but it was constant, and I got pretty tired of hurting by the time Thanksgiving came around.

When I would complain to Lisa—who is a Certified Nurse-Midwife, understand—her response was always the same. "You are fat. You eat too much. Your stomach is going to hurt until you lose weight." That's easy for her to say. She is a little-boned woman who eats all she wants and still has to run around in the shower to get wet.

My daughter, Jamie Leigh, was a little more helpful. Jamie is a Doctor of Pharmacy. Her mother and I spent a lot of money so the University of Georgia could teach her to sell drugs for a living. We have several kids at the school where I teach that can do that with no formal training whatsoever. Jamie suggested Gas-X or Alka-Seltzer.

I was familiar with Alka-Seltzer. I grew up watching my mama and daddy plop-plop and fizz-fizz after a big meal or a long night sitting around the kitchen table with their friends, swapping stories and drinking moonshine liquor. I also remembered Speedy Alka-Seltzer from the television commercials of my childhood and the "I can't believe I ate the whole thing—You ate it, Ralph" commercials from my youth. I had never tried Gas-X before, but I did now. I would have tried anything to get some relief from the pain in my stomach and sides.

Remember the old Jerry Clower story about the coon hunt? "Knock him out John! Oh! Shoot that thang!"

John Eubanks had climbed a tree to try to knock what he thought was a raccoon out of a tree, but wound up in an encounter with a bobcat. Jerry called it a "souped-up lynx." John kept begging his fellow hunters—I can't remember if Marcel Ledbetter was along or not—to shoot into the tree to kill the bobcat. The folks on the ground explained that they couldn't do that for fear of hitting John.

John finally pleaded, "Well shoot up here amongst us; one of us has got to have some relief!"

That's the way I was about my stomach, but no matter what I tried and how much or how little I ate, no relief was forthcoming. In the spirit of full disclosure, I will admit that we celebrated Thanksgiving, Christmas, New Year's and college football bowl season during this time, so any attempt I made at watching my food intake was half-hearted and futile at best.

Also in the spirit of full disclosure, there is no evidence whatsoever that the fall from the tree had anything to do with my pain and discomfort. In fact, I completely discount that theory because that would make me responsible for my own pain and suffering, and nobody wants to be held accountable for his own stupidity. At least I don't. But that's what Gary thought, and he could have been right. He often is—unless he is picking a horse in the Kentucky Derby or prophesying about the next elite Georgia quarterback.

At any rate, by January I had had enough and made an appointment with my internist, Dr. John Entrekin, to see if he could straighten me out. Dr. Entrekin, despite having graduated from Georgia Tech, might be my favorite doctor since J.B. Mitchell. Now understand, that is not to say anything against any of my doctors, past, present, or future. I just like Dr. John. He is mild-mannered and soft-spoken, and even though he is a serious runner and stays thin as a rail—and even though I wouldn't run if someone were chasing me and my weight always hovered around morbidly obese—he has never once fussed at me about my weight. He has pointed out that my obesity might kill me one day, but he has never fussed.

He is also one of the few doctors I have ever had who shared the gospel with me and testified about people he has known who have been healed by miracles that cannot be explained by medical science. But more about that conversation later. Bear with me now as I take a little detour to give you some background about doctors and me. I warned you in the prologue that the detours were coming. Feel free to skip over them if you like, but if you do, you'll miss some good stories and a significant moral or two.

Doctors and I go way back. One delivered me on March 10 in 1952, at the Porterdale hospital. The building is still there and sits atop Poplar Street, overlooking the entire north side of the village, including the site of the old school and the swimming pool. If my baby book can be trusted, and I can think of no reason it couldn't, I was delivered by Dr. Palmer and my mama stayed in the hospital a week. I weighed 6 pounds and 7 ounces and probably would have weighed more if Tommie Huckaby—my mother—had known not to smoke a pack of Winston cigarettes every day while she was carrying me. That's OK. I have more than overcome my low birth rate.

I have no personal recollection of the delivery, but I do remember going to see Dr. Palmer as a very young child. There were two rows of straight wooden chairs in his waiting room, situated back to back as if he might come out and organize a game of musical chairs at any moment. Dr. Palmer's nurse was Sarah Irwin, whom I would later know as Tootsie. That would be during my teenage years when her oldest daughter, Sally, and I would become close friends and I would spend an inordinate amount of time at her home. In the mid-1950s she was simply Dr. Palmer's nurse, but I liked her even then because she was full of personality and always teased me, in a good kind of way. She would come out into the waiting room and put a thermometer under everyone's tongue at the same time. Then she would come back and collect what she called the "glass cigarettes." Yes, times have changed.

That is the primary, and maybe the only, memory I have of the physician who brought me into the world. The first doctor I remember with great clarity is James B. Mitchell, the Bibb doctor during most of my childhood.

I suppose I should interject something here, just in case someone outside Newton County, Georgia, or someone younger than fifty ever reads this book. "The Bibb" refers to Bibb Manufacturing Company. Bibb owned all the houses in the little town of Porterdale, where I was raised, as well as all the property in the town and the three cotton mills that provided the livelihood of virtually all the residents of Porterdale and many residents of the adjoining counties.

The Bibb subsidized a doctor and a nurse for the mill hands and their families, and Dr. Mitchell was it when I was a child. His office was upstairs in a brick building across from the town post office. A long set of wooden stairs led to his office and I always climbed those stairs with dread. In the post-World War II '50s, doctors had one solution for what might ail a small boy. A penicillin shot was the solution to most medical problems and Dr. Mitchell only knew one place to jab a small boy with a hypodermic needle: right in the posterior.

We also had to go and see Dr. Mitchell for physicals every summer before we went to Scout camp—"we" being me and my fellow members of Troop 226. If I had known all of the dignity-defying examinations and procedures I would undergo once I was diagnosed with prostate cancer, I would have thought nothing of having to endure J.B. Mitchell instructing me to turn my head and cough.

I will never forget the first time my Scoutmaster, Booney Barnes, led me up those stairs for a pre-camp physical. I was scared to death, but Garry Sears, who was several years older than me, volunteered to go first when time came for short-arms inspection. The doctor chastised Garry and said, "That's a mighty weak cough." Garry responded, "Those are mighty cold hands."

I always think about that incident whenever any doctor gets anywhere near my private parts. But again, after what I have been through over the past two years, I no longer have any parts that can be considered truly private.

Dr. Mitchell made house calls, too. Any time I was too sick go to school, Mama would put me to bed and call Dr. Mitchell. I would stare glumly out the window, waiting for him to drive up and park his car on the street in front of the house. We didn't have driveways in Porterdale, we had back alleys. Dr. Mitchell didn't come to the back, however. He always walked right up to the front door.

His visits were short and sweet. He would listen to my chest with a stethoscope that was as cold as his hands. He would look in my ears and stick one of those wide wooden Popsicle sticks down my throat and make me say, "aah." Then he would have me roll over and would give me a shot. The worst part might have been the anticipation. He would put rubbing alcohol on a cotton swab and dab it around on my behind and then the stick would come without warning. Come to think of it, the stick was much worse than the anticipation.

To add insult to injury, he would always give my mother instructions to dose me once or twice a day with Castor oil. That was nasty stuff, but, again, it was nothing compared to some of the things I have ingested more recently.

One more doctor to tell you about before we get back to the cancer diagnosis.

When I was six, I was riding around my neighborhood on a tricycle. Now I could ride a two-wheeler when I was six, mind you, but somebody had stolen mine out of the back yard. Everybody knew who the family was who stole bikes in Porterdale. There were about a dozen kids in the family—maybe thirteen—and were the same people who always brought lice to school every year. Whenever that happened, every kid in the school had to hike across the street and up the stairs to Mrs. Annie Lee Day's office.

Mrs. Annie was Dr. Mitchell's nurse. She was one of the largest women I have ever known personally and had one of the most loving hearts. She loved everybody—especially every child who ever marched in front of her to receive an immunization of some sort or to have her pick through their hair looking for little critters. She used to go on all our class trips at the end of the school year. Sometimes we would go to places where swimming was available and we would marvel as Mrs. Annie—all 300-plus pounds of her—would float on top of the water and go to sleep.

Anyway, that's why I was riding a tricycle instead of a bicycle on the particular day in question. My bike had been stolen. A nylon cord had somehow become wrapped around the front axle of the trike, and it wouldn't go. I was trying to disentangle the cord and was pulling on it with all my might. The cord snapped and the tattered end flew back and hit me squarely in my left eye.

I went running down the street toward home, screaming bloody murder all the way. I actually thought I had been struck by a baseball hit by one of the older kids playing in a nearby yard. One of those kids—I think it was Pat Floyd—abandoned the game long enough to follow me home and tell my daddy what had happened.

Daddy picked me up and put me in our second-hand Buick and rushed me to Dr. Mitchell's office. He examined my eye and told Daddy that he had to get me to Atlanta immediately and find some-body who could save my left eye.

That somebody turned out to be a wonderful man named Dr. Dillard. This was 1958 and I fear his first name is lost to the ages, at least as far as I am concerned. All I know is how much my eye hurt and that I couldn't see anything out of it and that we had to drive to downtown Atlanta to the Doctor's Building on Peachtree Street every day for several weeks. Then we had to go twice a week. Then once a week. This went on for a long, long time.

I also know that I had to wear a black eye-patch for more than a year. This might seem like a pretty cool thing to have to do, giv-en the popularity of pirates these days. Surely you've seen Johnny Depp's portrayal of Captain Jack Sparrow. Trust me when I say that it is hard to be cool wearing overalls, brogan shoes with metal braces, and a buzz cut—which describes me in 1958. The eye patch was just one more source of torment, along with my big ears that stuck right out of the side of my head. My daddy's friend, Wyman Bowden, used to say that I looked like a '44 Ford coming down the road with both doors open.

The eye patch caused me considerable consternation when time came to register for first grade. There was no kindergarten for the little lintheads of my mill village. The principal, Jordy Tanner, took one look at me and told my mother that I couldn't learn to read prop-erly with one eye and that I would have to go back home and start school the following year when my eye had healed.

I was heartbroken because I had been looking forward to going to school for as long as I could recall. Through teary eyes, I told Miss Jordy that I could already read, that my father had taught me when I was four from the pages of the Atlanta Constitution. I am not sure if Jordy Tanner was from Missouri or not, but I had to show her that I could read before she would register me for first grade. She kept shoving different books of varying difficulty levels in front of me until I convinced her—my mother said after I successfully navigated a fourth-grade level book—that I could handle the academics at Porterdale School.

What caused my parents consternation was worrying about how they were going to pay Dr. Dillard. Every visit my daddy would ask about settling up the bill and every visit Dr. Dillard would answer, "I'm not worrying about the bill, I'm worrying about keeping this boy from going blind."

I suppose Dr. Dillard didn't have to worry about the bill because Homer Huckaby was worrying enough for both of them. My folks cut back on all spending, not that they spent that much to begin with, and saved every penny they could. After a year and a half of visits, Dr. Dillard finally declared my sight saved and announced that we didn't have to come back again.

My father insisted that the good doctor tell him how much we owed him and admitted that he might have to set up a payment plan. Dr. Dillard asked me to smile for him and I did. Then he looked at Daddy and said, "Is twenty dollars too much?"

I can't truthfully say that I remember it, but Mama always told me that we had the biggest steaks available in Atlanta for supper that night.

Back to Dr. Entrekin.

He gave me a thorough examination and had the nurse withdraw three or four vials of my precious blood from my throbbing veins. I am terrified of needles, and when this ordeal first began I could not have blood drawn without having three or four nurses holding my hands and fussing over me. I've had so much blood drawn now that I wouldn't care if Dracula himself came into the room with a big straw.

A few days after my visit to the doctor, his office called and made an appointment for me to come back in and discuss the findings. That wasn't very comforting because every other time I had blood drawn I got a recorded message informing me that everything was normal.

Nothing was normal about my blood that January, but neither was there anything that could pinpoint the unusual pain in my abdomen, which had not gotten any better despite the fact that I had actually begun a strict diet. I cut out all sweets, including iced tea and Coca-Colas. You know something is bad wrong when a good Southern boy stops drinking sweet tea for supper, and I do love my "Co-Colas," too.

I started eating whole wheat bread and cut out all meat except fish and chicken—usually baked or broiled. I ate a lot of green stuff that I had never eaten before. My general rule was, "if it tastes good, don't eat it."

When we met to talk about my blood work, Dr. Entrekin seemed very concerned about my pancreas and my liver. Some of the blood levels were in the abnormal range for both organs. I remember that he kept asking me over and over, in various ways, how much alcohol I consumed. That struck me as funny because I was a teetotaler until I was fifty, and now I never have more than one or two glasses of wine a month, and often go months at a time without imbibing so much as an ounce.

The doc admonished me from drinking anything at all for the next two weeks—I'm still not sure he ever really believed me when I assured him that I had not become the Conyers version of Otis Campbell overnight—and ordered another round of tests at the hospital. We are talking MRIs and x-rays and bone scans and nuclear tests and a colonoscopy. I had to swallow so much gross chalky liquid that I considered taking up the bottle in self-defense. Wherever they could find to poke a tube, they poked one. Whatever kind of machine they could find to hook me up to, they hooked me up to it. They had diagnostic stuff in that hospital that not even Dr. House has heard of—and still, the only thing they could find wrong with me was that my gall bladder might not be functioning quite right.

That was it. My second round of blood work did show improvement and Dr. Entrekin abandoned the plan I am certain he had formulated to send my away for 28 days, and instead sent me to a surgeon to discuss having my gall bladder removed. I was relieved to learn that I didn't have cirrhosis of the liver or pancreatic cancer or any of the other diseases that I had read about after Googling my symptoms on WebMD, but my stomach still hurt and nothing seemed to give me any relief.

I was ready to find a hunting party and beg them to "shoot up here amongst us," because I needed some relief.

Instead, I went to see a surgeon and scheduled a cholecystectomy. I was going to have my gall bladder removed.

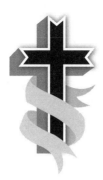

CHAPTER THREE

March has always been a great month for me. As previously reported, my first encounter with Dr. Palmer occurred in March and I have celebrated my birthday every March since. The state basketball tournament has been a part of the madness that is March for most of my life and March is when baseball players are in spring training. Daffodils and jonquils come out of hibernation and it is a great time to fly kites. I have always looked forward to March.

In 2011, not so much. The pain in my abdomen got worse and worse and worse. It was all I could do to get out of bed every day, and I am absolutely certain that my friends, family and co-workers just hated to be around me. Understand this, pain and I have never gotten along very well. I am not one of those stoic people who suffer along in silence when something is bothering them. I frown. I pout. I moan. I groan. And, worst of all, if somebody asks me how I am doing—I tell them. We all know that when someone asks, "How are you," they don't really want to know.

In other words, I was a big pain in the neck to be around—even more so than usual—and, truth be known, I was really a pain in a much lower extremity.

I said right up front that I wanted this book to be helpful to the readers, those who might be struggling with health issues and those who have never been sick a day in their lives. I am going to give you two pieces of advice here. It is completely free—except for whatever you paid for the book—and you may take it or you may leave it.

If you hurt, there is a reason you hurt. Somewhere out there is a doctor who can help you figure out why. Don't trust your diagnosis to friends who may have had, or who have known someone who has had, similar symptoms, and don't believe everything you read on the Internet. Secondly, don't feel guilty about sharing your burden with others. That's one of the most important lessons I learned through my ordeal.

Let me tell you how badly I felt as March approached. I didn't think I would live to see another one. I am not trying to be dramatic or elicit sympathy. I'm like Sergeant Joe Friday on the old Dragnet series. "Just the facts, ma'am, just the facts."

I am merely stating the facts.

I had mysterious pain everywhere. I had no energy. Some days I felt like my hair hurt. I also felt like poison was running all through my body. It was not a feeling I could describe, but I was as close to just shutting down as I had ever been in my life.

Since I was convinced that I would not see another March, I figured I would never have a chance to celebrate my birthday. So I decided to throw myself a party. I made a Facebook status inviting the world to my "Last Birthday Party."

We were going to have the party at Henderson's Restaurant in Covington, which is my very favorite place in all the world to eat, and it serves the best fried catfish, hushpuppies and sweet iced tea known to man—or woman, for that matter. To tell the truth, I was pretty chintzy. All I was going to provide was ice cream and cake, and folks who showed up were going to have to buy their own dinner. As it turned out, I am glad that was the plan because 104 people showed up, and even at Henderson's low prices, I couldn't afford to treat 104 people to dinner.

The large gathering gave my spirits a lift, but once the last bite of catfish was digested, I returned to my own little pity party and would often lie awake at night wondering what was wrong with me and why my doctors could not fix it. Sometimes I even remembered to pray for guidance, but I didn't really feel like I deserved an answer to my prayers.

At some point that winter, when I was in my deepest doldrums, Lisa and I drove down to Madison to enjoy a Friday night dinner with our friend Jolene who owns a little coffee shop and restaurant called

Perk Avenue. I don't think she is the same Jolene that Dolly Parton sang about, but if Dolly had ever met my Jolene, she probably would have. She's a wonderfully classy lady who makes all of the guests in her restaurant feel like guests in her home.

She came by our table that night and listened politely to my complaints and then listened to Lisa continue to blame every ailment I had—and some that I didn't—on my big belly. Jolene immediately walked back into her office and came out with a book solely dedicated to helping folks like me get rid of belly fat. I was willing to try anything at this point, so we borrowed Jolene's book and started my diet the next day—after filling up on her world-class steak and potatoes and cobbler, of course.

I don't know if it was the diet or an increased amount of exercise or the fact that I lost about twenty pounds over the next six weeks, but I began to feel better. I didn't feel quite right, understand, but I felt better. I felt so much better that the thought of being wheeled into an operating room and having one of my former students' father cut me open from stem to stern didn't appeal to me quite as much as it had a few weeks earlier when I had scheduled the operation. I called and cancelled.

Instead of spending my spring break recovering from surgery, I spent it, as usual, camping with friends and family at Jekyll Island. We rode bikes and sat around the campfire at night and played golf and ate copious amounts of seafood, just like we always had.

But this time wasn't like our other trips in the past. The bike riding made my rectum hurt so bad that I used a couple of tubes of Preparation H and a small jar of Vaseline that week. The seafood made me so bloated that my pain returned and I was no fun at all around the campfire. In other words, I was fairly miserable most of the week but tried my best to hide it, lest I make everyone in our rather large party just as miserable as I was.

When we got home from vacation, I thought things might calm down a bit, but they didn't. My pain steadily increased, the bloated feeling came back, and the mysterious pain in the walls of my side returned. Worst of all, I once again felt like poisons were flowing through my blood and I had no words to describe the feeling that made any sense to any of the medical or lay people with whom I talked.

I didn't know what to do about it because I had been through every examination anyone could think to give me. Plus, we were on the final leg of the marathon that is a school year for an AP teacher, and I didn't have time to do anything about my illness. I had to finish the semester with a strong push in order for my students to have any chance of passing the end-of-the-year Advanced Placement U.S. History exam. I decided to bide my time until summer, or at least until my annual physical examination that was scheduled for the middle of May. "Surely," I thought, "I can hold out another four weeks."

Right here I need to give the first of many shout-outs to my lovely wife, Lisa. I thought about not showing up for my physical. I had seen doctor after doctor and endured test after test. I gave considerable thought to just blowing off the appointment. I thought I would just call my surgeon back, plead temporary insanity, and ask if he would reschedule the surgery originally scheduled for March without another referral or examination.

When I discussed my plans with Lisa, reminding her that I was no longer morbidly obese, thanks to the belly fat thing I had done, she hit the roof, sent me to bed without any supper, and personally drove me to my physical the next morning.

It was a typical John Entrekin examination. He was positive and thorough. He asked me lots of questions about my pains and problems and, more importantly, listened to my responses without interruption or reaction. He, as always, apologized profusely before pulling on the dreaded rubber glove and asking me to drop my drawers and assume the position over his examination table. And no matter how hard I pleaded and no matter how many times I pointed out that I had undergone dozens of blood tests in recent months, he sent me to the lab so his nurses could hover over me and drain more of the precious serum from my veins.

He also admitted that he was just as frustrated with my situation as I seemed to be, and advised me to go ahead and have my gall bladder removed as soon as possible.

My surgeon was an understanding guy, but not understanding enough to schedule the surgery without another consultation.

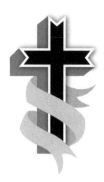

CHAPTER FOUR

The person who took out my gall bladder and stuck that ugly hernia that had been protruding from just right of my bellybutton for fifteen years was Dr. Andrew Harper. What I like most about him—other than the fact that he didn't botch my operation—is that while he is a very skilled and successful surgeon, he is as unpretentious as they come and introduces himself as Andy.

I taught all three of Dr. Harper's children and was his daughter's high school tennis coach. My kids were also in band with his kids, so naturally we had to spend a little bit of time catching up. I wish we had spent more time because after we had chatted one another up for a while, he informed me that before the surgery I had to have a lower GI series and then threw in an upper GI series for good measure.

I think the lower GI series might have been to punish me for waiting until June to have the surgery—or maybe it was another doctor who assigned that test. It is hard to remember when you've had as many procedures as I have. What I do remember about the lower GI is that I had to eat Jell-O and drink clear liquids for 48 hours beforehand. Jell-O and clear liquids—especially chicken and beef broth—would become a dietary staple for me over the next few months and I don't ever want to have either again.

Then there was the night before, which everyone agrees is the worst part. I don't know who might read this book and don't want to put images into anyone's head that might cause emotional distress—

or unrestrained laughter on the part of the reader if he or she ever happens to meet me in public—but I will say this: There is no dignified way to give oneself an enema and there is nothing fun about being tethered to the toilet all night. I promise you this, though. My insides were as clean as a whistle by the time I got to the hospital the morning of my test.

The upper GI was almost as bad because of the awful-tasting chalky goo they make you drink so much of. When all the tests were over and all was said and done, more was said than done.

What they found was a whole lot of adhesions around my esophagus and throughout my entire abdomen. I had scar tissue on top of scar tissue, which would create lots of complications for Dr. Harper and anyone else who might ever operate on me or consider operating on me.

I know. I know. You want to get to the part where you read about the cancer, but if I'm going to tell the story, I might as well tell it all, detours and all. I don't think it is a HIPAA violation if you reveal information about your own medical treatment.

I was 18 years old and bullet proof. I was a freshman at the University of Georgia and member of the varsity basketball team. I was the manager. The Southeastern Conference hasn't changed that much over the past forty years. I had my mother's car for the weekend and the world by the horns. One of my teammates, Charlie Anderson, needed a ride home to Macon. Like I said, I was 18 and bulletproof and had Mama's car—an Opel Kadett, which isn't a very big car to haul a six-foot, five-inch college hoops star around in.

I was going to drop Charlie off in Macon, understand, and didn't want to drive home alone, so I called my friend Carole Crawford, who was still in high school, and asked if she wanted to go along for the ride. Now you might wonder why Carole Crawford's mother would let her go on such a joy ride in the middle of the night, but I was one of those guys who every girl's mother really liked. The actual girls, not so much—but the mothers loved me and, more importantly, trusted me, so Carole's mother was more than agreeable.

We dropped Charlie off around midnight and headed back to Covington. We made it to Jackson, home of Fresh Air Barbeque, which is an institution in Georgia. I am certain that we were playing the radio at full blast and were probably laughing and talking about subjects that didn't amount to a hill of beans as we approached to turn off Highway 23 onto Highway 36, right in front of the Heart of Jackson motel. We had been riding parallel to a freight train and the last thing I remember was hearing the wail of its whistle as it approached a crossing just outside town.

The next thing I remember was being upside down in the car, lodged between the roof and the dash, the steering wheel crushing my chest. The next thing I remember after that was leaving the Jackson Hospital with my parents as dawn was breaking.

I will make a long story short right here. The trauma from the wreck did permanent damage to my esophagus. I had to leave school that spring to have surgery at St. Joseph's Hospital in downtown Atlanta. That was my first experience with a long-term hospital stay. I think my only other admission to a hospital was when I was six and had my tonsils removed.

Believe it or not, I remember that day very clearly. We drove up to the front of the old Newton County Hospital—what is now Newton Medical Center—and walked back to the operating room. My mama made me wear my pajamas to the hospital and I was embarrassed by that, even at age six. I carried my little stuffed elephant, which was my security blanket that nurse Annie Lee Day had given me as a baby.

They used ether as an anesthetic back then—thank you, Crawford W. Long—and I remember them putting that mask over my face and telling me to count backward from ten. I was six and hadn't started school yet. I couldn't count backward from two!

Somehow it all worked out. I woke up a little later and, like everyone else who was ever put to sleep by ether, threw up all over myself when I woke up. I also remember pitching such a hissy fit that the doctor let my mama take me home that afternoon and I didn't even have to spend the night in the hospital.

I did have a terribly sore throat, however, and had to eat Jell-O and drink chicken broth for several days. I must have had my tonsils out in the summer because I remember that tomatoes were coming in. Everybody else was having a tomato sandwich for lunch and I was having Jell-O for about the third or fourth straight day. I pitched another hissy fit and demanded to be allowed to have a tomato sandwich, too. Usually when I made demands I was sent outside to cut a switch, but I guess Mama felt sorry for me this time. Or maybe she just wanted to teach me a lesson. Either way, she let me have my way and made me a sandwich.

I still cringe when I think about that acidy tomato juice running down my still raw throat.

Now I know what you are thinking. You are thinking that a sixty-year-old man does not remember the details of his tonsillectomy at age six. Unfortunately, I do. I remember all sorts of things that happened long ago in minute detail. It is a blessing—and a curse. Of course, I can't remember where I put my car keys or what I had for breakfast this morning, but I can remember half-century ago in great detail. Sometimes I remember stuff that didn't even happen.

But back to St. Joseph's. It was April of 1971 and my room faced the back of the Regency-Hyatt House. That's the one with the blue domed revolving restaurant on top. At that time it was the tallest building in Atlanta—all 22 stories of it. I stayed there three weeks. It seemed like a year.

Without trying to get too technical, the wreck had straightened my esophagus. It no longer went into my stomach at an angle. At least that's how Dr. Newton Turk explained it to me. Everything that went into my stomach came right back up, into my mouth. Dr. Turk's solution was to scrape a bit of the material from the inside on my stomach and jerry-rig a valve that would allow food to go through my esophagus and into my stomach, but would not allow it to come back up.

I'm sure that was cutting-edge medical technology in 1971, and it worked, but I haven't been able to upchuck in 41 years and that has caused me a few problems over the years.

I must admit, my stay in St. Joseph's wasn't all bad. It was, and is, a Catholic hospital, of course. I had never met a nun before my stay there, but they were all over the place and came in and prayed for me several times a day. That gave me a lot of comfort. There were also a lot of young pretty nurses at St. Joseph's and I got a lot of attention from them.

I would have gotten a lot more attention from them if my boyhood friend—and sometimes nemesis—had not been in nursing school at Grady, just down the street.

Let me explain. I met Rosemary the summer before the fourth grade. Miss Martha Ramsey offered a summer enrichment program that summer for "smart kids." My mama signed me up for it and Rosemary, who was Miss Martha's niece, was in it, too.

We kind of liked one another right off the bat. She had beautiful brown eyes and dimples and a dark complexion. Miss Ramsey took us to the city greenhouse one day and the town gardener showed us how to repot petunias. I gave Rosemary the nickname "Petunia" that day and we were sweet on one another for the rest of that summer. I even got to visit her at Salem Campmeeting and hang out with the "tenters." That was a first for me. My family were regulars at Salem and always went to evening services, but until then I had never known what happened there during the daylight hours.

When school started I found myself in Mrs. Betty Robertson's class. Rosemary was in the class, too, of course. The only problem was that by then I was ready for my summer fling to be over. I wanted to go back to my regular girlfriend, Sylvia Hardegree. Yes, I was a fickle ten-year-old.

Rosemary wasn't about to let go so easy. I guess she knew a good thing when she saw it, and so for the next ten or twelve years we found ourselves in a love-dislike relationship. We would fight like cats and dogs at times and be best friends at times and even date at times—all the way up to and during college. It was complicated.

During the spring of 1971, Rosemary and I were in one of the off-periods of our on-and-off relationship—or at least I was. But my mother didn't know that, nor did she care. Her baby was in the hospital and Rosemary was in her first year of nursing school, which made her the same thing as a medical doctor in my mother's eyes, so she called Rosemary and asked her to check in on me. Boy, did she ever!

Almost every night, right after supper, Rosemary showed up. She was always so perky and I had a bad case of the mulligrubs throughout my hospital stay. I didn't feel perky and I didn't want to be around perky.

Besides, I felt awful and looked worse, and no 18-year-old wants to look and feel bad while an ex-girlfriend hovers about taking care of him—not even if that ex-girlfriend does date back to age ten.

Rosemary would shave me every day and—worst of all—brush my teeth for me. I was incapacitated, understand. I couldn't lift my arms or speak. I was defenseless. She would also pour baby powder onto my hair—which was nice and thick and lustrous at the time, although you would never guess that by looking at me now—and then spend a long time gently brushing the powder out of my hair.

I ask you, what could be worse than having a pretty young nursing student that you were trying to despise for reasons known not even to you, offer you that kind of treatment every day? I know, right?

In truth, the only reason I didn't like Rosemary coming to take care of me every night was the embarrassment factor because she did help make my confinement bearable. We would actually go out a few more times a year or so later. She eventually met a doctor, got married, moved to California and had three children. We saw one another about once a year after that—at Salem Campmeeting.

Rosemary died in 2003. I preached her funeral, in the Salem tabernacle.

There are other things I remember about my three weeks in St. Joseph's. About the third day after my surgery, for instance, the doctor came in to examine my incision, which was 10 inches long and ran right down the center of my chest. He decided that it was getting infected. He walked out of the room and came back and stuck a plastic toothbrush in my mouth and told me to clamp down on it and to hold onto the bed rails. Then he took a scalpel and sliced open the infected incision. My stomach popped open like an overripe watermelon.

Next, he had the nurse glue some white cloth contraptions to my sides. She poured Betadine down inside the cavernous opening in my chest, placed a wad of gauze pads over it, and laced the whole thing up like a pair of Converse All-Star high tops while I tried to bite through the toothbrush to keep from screaming in pain.

The doc explained that because of the infection, I would have to heal from the inside out. Every day for the next two months my bandage had to be changed. Now I have a souvenir of my experience that is about an inch wide in places, and when I go to the beach, mothers cover their children's eyes when I walk by.

I also recall the day the brand-new student nurse came in to give me a shot. I don't know what the shot was for, but I got them every day. This was near the end of my stay and I was feeling a little better, which meant I was feeling good enough to be grumpy and not quite so docile. Rosemary hadn't been by in a couple of days and I had a nice bit of stubble on my face. My hair was greasy due to lack of powdering and here was a young girl, not much older than me, getting ready to jab me with a needle. To make matters worse, she was perky.

She came over to the bed and asked, "How are we feeling today?" I hate it when nurses ask, "How are we feeling today?"

"I don't know how you are feeling," I growled at her, "but I feel like crap."

I don't think she responded to that remark, but I still remember the nervousness in her voice as she told me she was going to give me a shot. My arms felt like pin cushions by now so I rolled over and told her she had to give it to me in my hip. I don't think that is what she'd been hoping for.

To me, the worst part of getting a shot, as I said before, is the anticipation. Just like Dr. Mitchell used to do, this young Florence Nightingale-in-training poured alcohol on a piece of cotton and dabbed it on my butt. I tensed up, waiting for the stick. It never came. Instead she dabbed some more alcohol on my butt. I flinched and waited, again, for the jab that never came.

A third time she rubbed alcohol on me and finally I growled, "Would you give me the stupid shot, please!"

YEA THOUGH I WALK

She dropped her needle and ran out of the room. I never saw her again and have no idea if she ever got up enough nerve to give anyone a shot or not, but I bet she still remembers that day as clearly as I do.

The one other thing that sticks out in my mind about my stay in St. Joseph's Hospital is bedtime. Every night at 10:45, about fifteen minutes before shift change, my nurse would bring me a sleeping pill and a pain pill. I don't know what it was about that particular combination of medicine, but it would erase any and all inhibitions I might have had, and I would sit up in bed and begin to orate. I have no idea about the contents of my monologues, but I know that every nurse on the floor would come into the room and gather around my bed to hear them. One of the nurses told me that they lasted about ten minutes each time and that I would just conk out after that, in mid-sentence.

I think they hated to see me go.

Little did I realize that the complicated surgery I underwent at age 19 would rear its ugly head eleven years later—on my honeymoon.

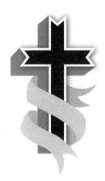

CHAPTER FIVE

I met the young woman who would become my lovely wife, Lisa, on March 30, 1981. I remember the date because it was the day John Hinckley Jr. shot Ronald Reagan. It was also the night that Indiana beat North Carolina to give Bob Knight his second NCAA basketball championship. A guy doesn't forget a day like that.

I was serving a two-year sentence teaching and coaching at Ravenwood Academy in Meigs, which is in deep south Georgia, way below the gnat line. Back in those days, teachers had to take real classes at real schools every five years or so to renew their certificates. I had almost allowed mine to expire and decided to grab a course at Valdosta State College, which was about ninety miles away.

Naturally I had to find a course that met my personal requirements. It had to be easy and only meet once a week—at night. I chose a first aid class taught by Dr. Nancy Scott. Although my roommate, Ken Cooper, who had failed that same course under Dr. Scott as an undergraduate at VSC, warned me that she was stern taskmaster, I decided to take my chances anyway.

After all, I was an Eagle Scout and had the First Aid merit badge. How hard could it be? Unlike my roomy, I intended to attend class, at least most Monday nights that semester.

I arrived at my class early and stood at the doorway, scanning the room and looking for the perfect place to sit. By perfect, I mean the desk next to the prettiest girl in class. I didn't have to look long.

There she was—third desk on the second row. She had long blonde hair that was brushed back and held in place by a special kind of band that made sexy little ridges in her hair. She had on a tight pink Izod polo shirt and short white shorts. Her legs went on for miles and she had a dark, dark tan. This was the Monday after Spring Break, understand.

There was a seat available right beside her, so I nonchalantly sat down next to her and tried to strike up a conversation. She wouldn't give me the time of day. I mean literally. I asked her for the time. She glanced at me and, noting that I was wearing a watch, suggested that I look at it.

Four-and-a-half months later, she asked me to marry her.

I said yes and the rest, as they say, is history. Which brings us to our honeymoon. We were married on December 18, 1982, on a Saturday night, one week before Christmas. We went to New Orleans on our honeymoon because that's where Scarlett and Rhett went for theirs. It was wonderful—for the first three days. On the fourth day, I started getting sick. I mean, really sick.

I woke up on a Tuesday, feeling perfectly fine. We had breakfast at Brennan's—I think I had Eggs Benedict and Bananas Foster for dessert. I am relatively sure it was the first time I'd ever had dessert with my breakfast, and I am absolutely certain it was the first time a waiter ever set fire to my breakfast dessert right there at my table.

For lunch we stopped in at Felix's and I had a dozen oysters on the half shell. If you've never been to Felix's Restaurant & Oyster Bar in the French Quarter in New Orleans, you need to put that on your to-do list. The atmosphere is second only to the food. The first dozen oysters were so tasty that I had two more—dozen.

As we were getting ready to go out for supper that evening, I began to have a little stomach ache, which wasn't surprising, considering all the gastronomical challenges I had given my stomach that day. What was surprising was that I could barely eat my supper at the Court of Two Sisters, and I am the one who asked Lisa if we could go back to the hotel and turn in early. During most of our stay she had been the one who had to pull me away from Bourbon Street every night.

The pain in my stomach grew worse with each passing minute. I felt like I needed to throw up, but that was not an option for me because of the valve the doctors had inserted into my esophagus when I was in college. Nothing would come out the other end either—and if you think that is distasteful to read, imagine being the one to write about it—from memory!

I tossed and turned and moaned and groaned all night, and if Lisa had been real smart she would have tried for an annulment as soon as government offices opened for business the next morning. Instead, since I still wasn't willing to think about food, much less eat any, she ordered room service for herself for breakfast and then we went for a tour of the Louisiana Superdome.

I was a gamer. I really was. I tried to keep a smile on my face, but I could not walk past a restroom without going in and trying to find some relief from my bloated, aching stomach. I probably sat on just about every toilet in the building, all to no avail.

Our plans had been to visit the horse track after the stadium tour so that is what we did. It was Lisa's first horse race. I tried to explain the racing form to her and showed her how to make bets. While she went to place a two-dollar bet on the first race of the day, I sprawled out across one of the bleachers and prayed that someone would kill me and take me out of my misery. Lisa's horse came in first and she won twelve bucks. She wanted to spend the rest of the week at the horse track but I had had enough. I pleaded with her to walk me outside the track and find a cab.

We went back to our hotel and I spent the next few hours sprawled across the bed. I am not sure what all patent medicines Lisa gave me, but I do know that every time I smell Pepto-Bismol to this day, I have an urge to eat raw oysters. She walked me around the room. She had me soak in a hot bath. Nothing eased the pain. Finally, around 5 p.m., I had had all I could stand. "We've got to get to a hospital," I told my bride of about a hundred hours.

Now understand, Lisa was barely 21 and a senior in college. She had never traveled anywhere on her own and there we were in a great big city, married to an old man whose life seemed to be ebbing out of him because of eating too much rich Creole and Cajun cuisine. It must have been a nightmare for her.

We made our way down to the front desk and asked one of the clerks how to get to the nearest hospital. He started trying to direct us to Charity Hospital. His partner, who seemed a bit more aware, insisted that we go to the Hotel Dieu, which wasn't a hotel at all but a very fine Catholic hospital, which happened to be right across the expressway from the same Superdome we had visited that morning. That morning seemed to have occurred in another lifetime by then.

The clerk sent a valet to bring our car around and then went outside himself and hailed a taxi. Lisa walked me out to the street, and together she and the helpful desk clerk poured me into the car. The clerk instructed the cab driver to lead us to the Hotel Dieu, and admonished him to drive slowly so Lisa could keep up with him in the rush hour traffic.

Richard Petty couldn't have done a better job of weaving in and out of traffic and keeping the nose of our brand new Chevy Monte Carlo on the cab driver's bumper. When we got to the hospital, the cabby blew his horn and waved good-bye, leaving us to try and figure out where to go. We pulled up into the emergency room entrance and two men in business suits who seemed to be just getting off work walked up to the car to offer assistance. They took one look at me and one of the men ran into the emergency unit and hurried back with a wheelchair.

The other man found someone to park our car and they hurried me right into the ward. We didn't stop at the admissions desk to give our names. Nobody asked us for an insurance card. They just wheeled me right into the back and stretched me out on one of those rolling stretchers. Two minutes later, a doctor appeared from nowhere and started examining me and asking Lisa about my symptoms. He started doing percussion on my stomach as he listened through his stethoscope

"When's the last time you had a bowel movement?" I remember him asking. I admitted that it had been about three four days ago—when I was still single.

"When's the last time you vomited?" he asked next.

"1971," I told him.

He turned to Lisa and said, "He has a bowel obstruction." He could have told her I had a bilateral-whatchamacallit-doohickey and it would have made just as much sense to me. I had never heard of a bowel obstruction, much less had one. The doc called for an NG tube, whatever that is, and the next thing I knew he really and truly was going down my nose with a rubber hose—right into my stomach.

I don't know exactly what the nurse did to prime that siphon, but the next thing I knew, the vilest, smelliest green goop that I had ever seen was pouring out of my stomach, up through that tube and out my nose. There seemed to be gallons of the stuff.

Then they gave me a shot that sent me to Sleep City faster than you can say ether. When I came to, I was in a hospital room with a great big window. My view overlooked the Superdome where the Georgia Bulldogs would be showing up in about eight days to play Pittsburg with the National Championship on the line. Lisa was right by the bed looking really worried, which is unusual for her.

"Sorry you said 'I do?'" I asked, expecting her to rush over, grab my hand and say, "Oh, no! Of course not."

What she said was, "I'm not sure yet," and then asked how much life insurance I had.

The doctor interrupted that poignant moment and gave the hard, cold facts. I can't recall the entire conversation, but the pertinent points were that I did indeed have a bowel obstruction, and if we'd waited a couple of hours later, my bowels would have perforated and Lisa would have been the prettiest widow at Valdosta State College that winter semester.

I needed an operation and I needed it immediately. I do remember my response to that news.

"How long will I be in the hospital?" I asked.

"Ten days to two weeks," was the honest reply.

I looked out the window at the Superdome, imagining the red tide that would be surrounding that building on New Year's Day. Then I looked at Lisa, who looked like she had the weight of the world on her narrow young shoulders.

"Nothing doing," I said. "We'll drive home and have the surgery there."

"Can't," insisted the doctor. "You might make a nine-hour drive without incident or your intestine might burst and you could die in the car before you found a hospital."

"What if we fly?" was my next question.

The doctor frowned, and gave careful thought to what I had said. "How far from the airport in Atlanta is it to your hospital?" he asked.

"Thirty minutes."

The doc hesitated. "The problem," he finally said, "is that you need your IV, you need your morphine and you need the NG tube that is draining your stomach. It's doubtful the airlines would accept you with all that stuff unless you were traveling with a nurse."

"I'm a nurse!"

Everybody in the room looked at Lisa. I was shocked by her proclamation because she was not, in fact, a nurse. She was a senior in nursing school, but she was not a Registered Nurse and would not be for several more months.

She fooled the doctor, though. He looked us over and decided that we might actually be able to make it onto a plane if the angels who protect children and fools were with us. They were.

Everybody got busy. The doctor left and started making phone calls to Dr. Millard Ross in Conyers in preparation of handing off his patient. Lisa had to leave the hospital, drive back to our hotel in the French Quarter, pack up all our luggage and drive back to the hospital. Somebody had to make flight reservations—for tickets that would have to be purchased with cash, because in 1982, neither of us had a credit card.

That brought up another problem. It was just a few hours before Christmas Eve and all the flights between New Orleans and Atlanta were full. Our doctor eventually called Delta and explained our situation. Consequently, two poor souls got bumped from their flight for our medical emergency. I hope Delta hooked them up with free passes to Hawaii or something for their trouble.

I wasn't aware of any of that, though. I was enjoying the morphine drip flowing into my arm, and after I was certain the doctor wasn't going to try to keep us hostage in New Orleans until Herschel Walker arrived, I just dozed off.

The next thing I recall was being pushed out to the car in a wheelchair and dumped in the front seat. I still had all sorts of tubes—in my arm, in my nose; stuff going in, stuff coming out, into a clear plastic bag. I was a sight.

I also remember that we only had a short time to make the flight and a long ride to the airport. Just as we started to get on the expressway, a Louisiana state trooper shut down the ramp for a funeral precession.

At least he started to. Lisa rolled down the window, ready to cry if she had to, although that's something she doesn't do, and shouted, "I have to get my husband to the airport!"

The trooper took a look at me, slumped over in the car and stopped the funeral. "I think there is still a little hope for this guy," he said. "Let's let them go first."

Our car was still decorated, by the way, from the wedding with "Just Married" and all other sorts of slogans scrawled all over the windows and back deck. We were going to leave the car at the airport.

We parked our car and somehow made our way inside. A Delta Red Coat brought a wheelchair and rolled me right up to the ticket counter. Luckily they were expecting us and, even more luckily, terrorists had not thought to fly airplanes into buildings yet and there was no security checkpoint to navigate.

They rushed us to the gate where they were awaiting our arrival. Everyone looked at us with great curiosity as the gate agent walked me down the aisle to our seats. Our assigned row was three seats wide and a lady was sitting on the outside seat. She shot us a horrified glance and tried to move over to the window seat, but this was Lisa's first time on an airliner and she wanted to sit by the window. We crawled over the poor lady, apologizing profusely. Lisa sat by the window and I sat in the middle, green yuck still pouring through the tube sticking out of my nostrils into the bag, IV needle still stuck in my arm.

YEA THOUGH I WALK

The poor lady scrunched as far as she could toward the aisle and tried hard not to look at me. Finally, having seen more than she could stand, she called the flight attendant over and said, "Miss, could I please have a different seat? I think I'm bothering him."

Lisa assured her that I had just had a great big dose of morphine before leaving the hospital and that nothing in the world would bother me. At first, the attendant explained that the plane was full and there were no other seats. Then she took pity on the woman and offered to let her sit on the jump seat in the back of the plane.

Honesty compels me to admit that I do not remember the flight or arriving in Atlanta or anything else for twenty-four hours. The next thing I remember is waking up on Christmas Day in a hospital room, surrounded by my parents and new in-laws and most of Lisa's family. They were a grim-looking bunch.

It was decided that when Christmas was over, Lisa's brother and his girlfriend would fly out to New Orleans and drive my Monte Carlo home. They said they got a lot of strange looks when they showed up, three days later, to claim the "Just Married" car that had been abandoned the night before Christmas Eve.

I later learned by talking to my surgeon, Millard Ross, that my bowel obstruction was caused by scar tissue left behind by the doctors who did my esophageal stricture operation, all those many years ago. He also warned me that he had left behind scar tissue, too, and that it was a matter of when, not if, they would cause me problems.

The "when" was in June and August of 2011—but we aren't quite there yet.

There is one little aside that I feel compelled to share because I don't believe in coincidences, but I do believe greatly in God-incidences.

When we crossed the state line into Louisiana, on our way to New Orleans, we stopped at the Welcome Center. We were stretching our legs, looking at the folders advertising nightclub tours and cheap hotels when a nice lady who worked at the center approached us and asked if we were on our honeymoon. When we assured her we were, she asked where we were staying. I told her and she said, out of the blue, that she could get us a nicer room at the Holiday Inn

Chateau LeMoyne. She assured us that is was just as nice as the hotel I had booked and we could save $360 by staying there.

Now understand, we didn't have a lot of money. I was a teacher and coach at Clarkston High School and always spent just a little more than I made each month. Lisa was still in college. Every penny counted and I had budgeted our honeymoon right down to the penny—and we only dealt in cash in those days. A $360 savings would be huge. We graciously accepted the lady's offer.

I told you that to tell you this. When we bought our airline tickets at the New Orleans airport for our emergency flight to Atlanta, they were exactly $180 each—$360.

God is good, all the time. All the time, God is good.

We spent Christmas in the hospital and the week after Christmas in the hospital and went home on New Year's Eve. Lisa took good care of me and I realized that when she stood at that altar and promised to stand with me "for better or for worse, and in sickness and in health," she wasn't just whistling "Dixie."

Now I had two really cool parallel scars running down the front of my chest. I never gave another thought to the adhesions growing in my chest wall—until my final pre-surgery appointment with Dr. Andy Harper.

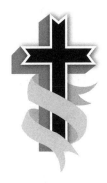

CHAPTER SIX

Adhesions and scar tissue and the discussion thereof would dominate my life for the next several months—and not in a good way. When I went back to see Andy Harper for my final briefing before the gall bladder surgery, which we scheduled for June 1 so I wouldn't miss a single minute of the riotous fun that shutting down another school year brings, he was direct and to the point and pulled no punches.

"This is going to hurt," he told me. "It's going to hurt a lot and for a while."

I stupidly nodded my head, thinking that I was actually comprehending what he was saying.

"The operation is going to hurt," he repeated. "It's not going to hurt a little bit. It's going to hurt a whole lot." He emphasized *whole lot.*

"Did I mention that it is going to hurt," he asked for a third time. I started laughing then, not because I was looking forward to the pain, but because he reminded me of Jesus asking Simon Peter if he really loved him, when they met at that fish fry after Jesus had already been crucified but was yet to ascend into heaven.

After we had agreed that the surgery—and the recovery—was going to hurt, Dr. Harper reminded me that the removal of the gall bladder might ease the pain in my abdomen and that it might not. I got the idea that he didn't want to be made the fall guy in a ruthless post-op newspaper column penned by yours truly.

Then we had to discuss the adhesions. "You know," he reminded me, "when we did your upper GI we saw a lot of adhesions and a lot of scar tissue. I am hoping to do this surgery laparoscopically, but there may be too much scar tissue to do that."

I just nodded. I really didn't know any other way to respond.

He went on. "I won't know until I get in there whether I can do it with the laparoscope or not, and if I can't, I'm not going to wake you up and ask you what you want to do. I'm going to go ahead and cut."

I nodded again. I was getting good at that.

"OK," he said. "But if I have to cut, you will be in the hospital for a few days and you will have to have a catheter."

I had already told him that I would do anything to avoid a Foley catheter, which is a flexible tube that is passed through the urethra and into the bladder in order to allow urine to drain into a collection bag outside the body.

Not to be too graphic, but the dude was going to stick a rubber hose down my penis and catch my pee in a bag. I wanted no part of that and said a silent prayer, right then and there, that Dr. Andy Harper would be able to perform my surgery laporascopically. I am positive that this organ was designed strictly for one-way traffic.

After I assured him that I knew I was in for a lot of pain that might or might not ease my discomfort and that I might have to be cut open, I signed all the paperwork and we said our goodbyes. The next step was to show up at Newton Medical Center, where I had spent my honeymoon 29 years earlier, and take care of all my pre-certification paperwork.

I did that on a Friday afternoon, May 27. I had a bit of a problem at the hospital because as I sat outside and waited for my name to be called to the lab to get my blood drawn and whatever else they were going to do to me, it seemed every single person in Newton and Rockdale County, those I knew and those I did not, walked past me—and every single one was nosey as the devil and demanded to know *why I was there and what they were going to do to me.*

The nurse didn't ask such personal questions when she was recording my medical history.

Finally, my friend Joyce peeked out of her office and realized my plight. She took me back into a private office and told me that I could wait my turn there, out of the glare of the public spotlight. Remember those God-incidences I mentioned earlier? This was another one, because about two minutes after Joyce had provided me with some much-needed privacy, my cell phone rang—or beeped or buzzed or vibrated or whatever it is that cell phones do these days. I looked down to see who was calling, and John Entrekin's name came up. I didn't take that as a positive sign. Rarely do doctors call patients on their cell phones. It is rarer still when they call on their personal phones on a Friday afternoon.

I answered anyway.

We exchanged pleasantries and he asked me where I was and what I was doing. I told him that I was at the hospital waiting for the pre-cert for what I considered the mother of all surgeries. Dr. Harper had warned me that it was going to hurt! Remember?

Then Dr. John told me that he had some news that would take my mind off the surgery for a while. "Oh?" I asked. "What's that?"

"I am afraid you have prostate cancer."

I don't know how long I sat there, silently staring at my phone. How long did you sit still in the movie theater once you realized that Walt Disney was going to let Old Yeller die? How long do you sit in a football stadium after the other team wins the game with a last-second field goal? It might have been a minute or two or it might have been just a couple of seconds.

"Prostate cancer?" I finally got out.

"Yes, I'm sorry. Your PSA went from nothing at all to 6.0 over the past five months. It could just be an enlarged prostate but everything felt normal during your examination last week and that is a sharp rise in a short period of time. I want you to go ahead and make an appointment with the urologist as soon as possible. We need to get a biopsy."

I thanked Dr. Entrekin for letting me know as soon as possible. He was right, too. His news did take my mind off the pre-cert. I walked through that procedure like a zombie. My gall bladder and hernia and whatever else Dr. Harper was going to do were the least of my worries.

"OK. You've got this," I said to myself. "Be stoic. Be tough. Stiff upper lip, as the British say."

Then I began to tell myself all those lies I had heard over and over and over—the same lies all my friends would be telling me soon.

"If you're going to have cancer, prostate cancer is the best kind to have."

"More men die with prostate cancer than from it."

"It's a piece of cake."

It just so happened that Lisa and I were going away for the Memorial Day weekend. My friend Bill Tanner, who was the head honcho at Amicalola Falls State Park in Northeast Georgia, had invited us to spend the weekend at the lodge and do a book signing. We were looking forward to getting away for a few days before my upcoming surgery. When I walked into the house, Lisa was standing in the kitchen, holding her overnight bag.

I suppose I had a strange look on my face—stranger than usual, I mean—because Lisa took one look at me and asked, "What's wrong?"

I took a deep breath and said, "Dr. Entrekin called and said that I have cancer."

Then, despite all the promises I had made to myself on the drive home from the hospital, the tears came. It wouldn't be the last time, not by a long shot.

That weekend is still a bittersweet blur in my mind. We had promised ourselves that we would stay as disconnected from the outside world as possible during our getaway. That didn't mean no cell phones, but I did leave my laptop computer at home, which is something I never, ever do.

The lodge at Amicalola is beautiful and the setting is spectacular, with giant glass walls providing a most excellent view of the Appalachian foothills. The lodge is positioned so that most rooms provide a view of the sun setting over those same mountains.

Being Memorial Day weekend, the lobby of the lodge was decked out in red, white, and blue, and there was an impressive display that hit my eye as I walked into the door that featured an old bomber jacket and some black-and-white photographs of military heroes from a bygone era. Upon closer examination, I realized that one of the clear-eyed young men staring back at me from one of the pictures was my old friend, Dr. Terrell Tanner, Bill's dad.

Dr. Tanner had been my team doctor when I was a young football coach at Cousins Middle School in Newton County, and he was one of our school's best supporters. I had been Bill's P.E. coach there and his sister Sarah's teacher. We were having old home week in the mountains and I was learning a lot of things I didn't know about my friends. That was a good thing and provided a distraction. I needed every distraction I could get.

I also met a lot of very nice people who stopped by to look at my books. Some of them even bought a couple. One day a ranger came by the lodge and brought a few birds of prey with her, and we learned about owls and eagles and falcons and hawks. Another day she brought a bag of snakes, and I learned how to stay away from snakes. I am certain that every single reptile I have ever encountered has been a cottonmouth water rattler.

Most of all we hiked. There are beautiful trails all over Amicalola Falls, including the approach trail that leads to Springer Mountain and the southern terminus of the Appalachian Trail. We ran into a couple of greenhorns who thought they might walk all the way to Maine. I was certain they wouldn't make it out of the park.

Being near the AT and hiking up and down the rugged trail next to the falls, which the Cherokee Indians called "dancing waters," brought back fond memories of my younger days in the Boy Scouts. I had spent a lot of time walking those trails, and it seemed a bit ironic that I would be there that weekend as I began to contemplate the life I had lived and the life I had before me. I can't say if hearing the words, "I am afraid you have cancer," has the same effect on everyone, but it certainly had that effect on me.

I was determined not to make a big deal out of my disease, especially until we learned for certain that I did indeed have cancer, but I couldn't quite get it out of my mind, either. So we walked and talked and laughed and wondered what the future held while giving thanks for the many blessings we had already received in life. And make no mistake; I had received more than my share—more than any ten people's share—of blessings in my life.

First of all I was fortunate enough to have been born and raised in Porterdale. I had the best childhood anyone could ever imagine. I had two parents who loved me unconditionally and made sure I knew right from wrong. They kept books in our house and made me mind my teachers and kept up with my schoolwork. They loved me enough to hug me when I needed it and spank me when I needed it, and were always wise enough to realize when I needed which.

The kids who were raised in Porterdale in the 1950s and '60s were the luckiest kids on earth. We had great schools with excellent teachers, first-class athletic facilities with a pool and a gym and ball fields, and we had the run of the village. We could be out the door as soon as it was daylight and didn't have to be home until our mamas called us for supper.

None of us had much money, but we didn't realize that. We had plenty to eat and each of us had what everybody else had. It really was an idyllic place to live.

When I graduated from high school and matriculated at the University of Georgia—hallowed be thy name—I took sociology. My professor learned that I was from Porterdale and announced to the class, "Mr. Huckaby was raised in poverty, in a north Georgia mill village."

My professor was obviously educated far beyond his intelligence. We weren't poor in Porterdale, we just didn't have much money. There is a big difference, let me tell you.

I graduated from Georgia, which was another blessing, and had a lovely wife and three of the best children a man could possibly hope for. I had been everywhere and done everything, and I spent a great deal of my weekend walking the trails and counting those blessings. But I would be less than honest if I didn't admit that I spent a lot of time wondering about the future and beating back tears, too. Like I said, the weekend was bittersweet and was a prelude to what would be a very traumatic two weeks.

I had a little bit of time to sit and visit with Bill Tanner, and I allowed myself to share the news about my cancer with him. He was very encouraging and was, I believe, the first person to promise to pray for strength to fight that particular battle. I am certain he has kept his word and I am even more certain that he has gained legions of fellow prayer warriors since that May weekend.

We came back from the mountains on Monday evening. I spent all day Tuesday fasting, in preparation for the next day's surgery, and scouring the Internet for every bit of information I could find about prostate cancer.

I didn't like what I found.

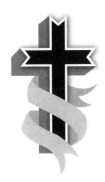

CHAPTER SEVEN

We liked watching the television show, Monk, at my house. For the uninitiated, Monk was a quirky little television show starring Tony Shalhoub about a neurotic police detective who could solve any murder San Francisco could throw at him but who had trouble coping with everyday life. When asked about his almost psychic investigative genius, Monk, the title character, would always say, "It's a gift—and a curse."

That pretty well describes the Internet, at least when you start trying to research a medical condition, real or imagined. There is a wealth of information out there—a wealth of really good, pertinent, and scientifically proven information. There is also a ton of garbage that will scare you death if you pay attention to it.

Every medical professional I have encountered since my fight with cancer began has advised me to stay away from the Internet. I have advised everyone I know over the years to avoid diagnosing his or her own medical problems over the Internet. So has my lovely wife, Lisa, who is a Certified Nurse Midwife.

And everyone I know, as soon as they get the first lump or bump or cough or cold or sign of a rash, logs onto the World Wide Web and places themselves at death's door before they log off the computer.

I am no exception, and I spent the entire day before my gall bladder surgery reading about prostate cancer. I learned more than I ever wanted to know. Some of it even turned out to be true.

YEA THOUGH I WALK

When I first Googled "prostate cancer," the search engine turned up 58 million hits in sixteen seconds. I am a fast reader and I had all day, but I still couldn't read 58 million commentaries and articles about prostate cancer in one day. I decided for the time being to stick to the ones concerning testing and diagnosis, since I really didn't know for sure that I had it.

Most of the articles I did read were quite unsettling.

Much of it was just basic information. The prostate is a walnut-sized gland. It is part of the reproductive system and wraps around the urethra and yada, yada, yada … I knew all of that. I had read it the previous year when my father-in-law, who was in his mid-seventies, was diagnosed with the same disease. I was reading a lot closer this time, however, because now it was my body that cancer was trying to overtake.

I found out that prostate cancer is the leading cause of death in men over the age of seventy-five. I wasn't yet sixty. I rationalized that if I made it fifteen more years I really couldn't kick too much.

I also read a lot about the risks factors to try and decide why this particular malady was plaguing me. It turns out that African-American men are at a higher risk than Caucasians and that the disease was a bigger threat in men over sixty. I read about several other risk factors that did not apply to me.

For instance, I didn't have a brother or father with prostate cancer. I have never smoked cigarettes or abused alcohol and I am not a farmer and I have never worked in a tire plant. I'm serious. Those were listed as high-risk occupations, although I have no idea why. I was feeling pretty good and even began to think that maybe Dr. Entrekin was mistaken and that I simply had an infection of some sort. Then, uh oh!

Men who eat a diet high in animal fat are at major risk, according to what I found on the Internet. Lord, help us. That would be everybody I grew up around and every Southerner worth his salt. When I was growing up I ate bacon and eggs and country ham and sausage—or some combination thereof—every morning for breakfast. At night I ate fried chicken and country fried steak and ham and pork chops. I'm not trying to make you hungry. I'm just telling you what I ate.

Not much has changed about my diet. I just shook my head. If eating a lot of meat gives you prostate cancer, I knew that I had earned every bad cell I had. Of course, there are probably vegetarians that have the disease, too, so I didn't beat myself up too much about the billion or so calories I have ingested in my lifetime.

Next I looked at the symptoms and couldn't figure out if I had any of them or not. Many of them seemed to deal with a man's urinary habits, but every sixty-year-old man I know has to go a lot more often than they used to and none of my friends sleep through the night anymore—especially to hear their wives tell it. Leaking or dribbling at the end of your stream can be a symptom, too.

Reading that one made me smile and think about my high school chemistry and physics teacher, Joe Croom. Croom was about the best teacher I ever had and one of the best people I have ever known. He was also our Key Club advisor. In those days Key Club was strictly for boys. He used to have a little poem about going to the bathroom. He said you could "beat it and shake it, hit it on the wall, but put it in your pants for the last drop to fall."

So, yes, I had most of those symptoms, but so did every other male I knew over the age of fifty.

Then I read that pain in the bones, particularly the lower back or pelvis, could be a symptom of cancer and could also indicate that the cancer had spread. That alarmed me because I did have pain in my back, pelvis, and ribcage, but I had just assumed that was from growing old.

The next article I read was all about the PSA test. It was my PSA score that had alarmed my doctor in the first place. PSA stands for prostate-specific antigen, which is, apparently, a protein produced by prostate cells. The more of these antigens in a man's blood, the higher the likelihood of cancer. I learned that a high number doesn't always mean cancer but I also learned that another major indicator is how rapidly the PSA is rising.

At any rate, for a man my age, the safe range should have been below 2.5 and I was a 6—and I had gone from 0 to 6 in about five months. The more I read, the more discouraged I got. By the time I was ready for bed, I had convinced myself that I had the most severe case of cancer anyone had ever had. I tried my best to put the whole thing out of my mind because there was nothing I could do until I had the biopsy and learned the results of that test. Besides, I was having major surgery the next morning and would have no idea whether that surgery would be open or laparoscopic until after the deed was done.

I pretended I was Scarlett O'Hara and said to myself, "I will think about that tomorrow. After all, tomorrow is another day."

Then I took an Ambien and went to sleep.

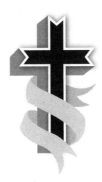

CHAPTER EIGHT

Dr. Andy Harper proved to be a man of his word. After the surgery, I hurt. I didn't hurt a little bit; I hurt a lot—and I hurt a lot for a while.

There was good news, however. I woke up from the surgery in one of those reclining chairs in the recovery room instead of a bed, which meant that Dr. Harper had been able to skillfully cut through and around all the adhesions in my chest and abdomen to remove my gall bladder without slicing me wide open. That is significant because there was no tube and no collection back dangling from my privates. Praise the Lord.

He had also managed to fix the hernia that had been poking out of my belly like a big sore thumb for a dozen years. I was excited. Now I could stroll up and down the beach without a t-shirt and my only embarrassing projection would be my enormous belly itself. While he was at it, Dr. Harper told me that he cut through a lot of the adhesions that had been binding the inner muscles of my abdomen and chest in hopes that more of the unexplained pain in that area would be relieved.

It was win, win, win—except that I would hurt like the devil for weeks. But I couldn't say that I hadn't been warned.

My surgery was on a Wednesday and I was instructed to take it easy until the following Tuesday when I would report to my local urologist for my prostate biopsy. Six days is a long time for me to take it easy. I was so groggy Wednesday night when I got home from the hospital that I slept in my recliner all night. Pharmaceuticals helped.

Thursday, I lay around moaning and groaning and generally making a nuisance of myself. Lisa was a good sport and waited on me hand and foot for about two hours. After that it was, "Get up and get it yourself. You need to move around."

On Friday, I felt worse than I had on Thursday, if that were possible. Friday night, however, there was work to be done. Our dear friend, Diane Howington, was hosting a charity event—a trivia contest, of all things—and had enlisted my help many months before.

Diane is a great person with a heart as big as Texas. We met when "we had our first child together." Her words, not mine—but I can't let that go without an explanation.

Diane Howington's grandfather was Gailey Summers, who owned Gailey's Dry Goods and later Gailey's Shoes in Olde Town Conyers. When Lisa and I were expecting our first child, who turned out to be a precocious little girl we named Jamie Leigh, Lamaze classes were all the rage. If you want to know all about Lamaze classes, go to YouTube and listen to Bill Cosby's bit. He's a lot funnier than I could ever be. But back to Diane.

She and her husband, Mark, were expecting their first child, too. They would also have a little girl they named Marci. To make a long story short, we became lifelong friends. We have raised our kids together and laughed and cried together and developed a Salem Camp Meeting relationship as well as a personal one. We are practically family, in other words.

I have never heard Diane ask anybody for anything for herself, but when it comes to helping others, she is not a bit shy and will ask anybody for anything on behalf of someone who needs food or a place to live or a second chance at life. It's her nature and one of her spiritual gifts so it didn't matter to her that I was only forty-eight hours removed from the surgeon's scalpel. She needed her trivia questions read and had drawn a big crowd to her event based on the promise that I would be reading them. So when Friday night came, I popped a couple of Percocets and, accompanied by Lisa, Jamie, and my son, Jackson, I went to Diane's event and read trivia questions.

Most of the crowd wished I had stayed home. They said my questions were too hard. I don't think so, but I'll let you decide. Let me share a couple of them.

Question: What major party's presidential candidate ran for election by passing out campaign literature that read, "AU-H2O?"

It was Barry Goldwater. Who wouldn't know that?

Question: What was Wally Pipp's claim to fame?

OK. Maybe that was a hard one for a young crowd. He was the person Lou Gehrig replaced when he began his record-setting streak of 2,130 consecutive baseball games. I know Cal Ripken has since broken the streak, but Gehrig will always be the real Iron Horse to me.

One more. Where is the Sea of Tranquility?

Give up? It's on the moon.

So maybe my questions were a bit hard, but old folks like me would have known most of them. Grady Duke's team won and one of the prizes was a party for eight at Hooters. He promised he would invite me, but he didn't.

Sorry for the detour, but everybody should know about Diane.

My summer was, in a word, miserable. It took me a long time to get over the pain from the gall bladder and hernia surgery. It also took me a long time to get used to not having a gall bladder. I don't eat the blandest diet in the world, understand, and willpower and I have never been one a first-name basis. In fact, we are virtual strangers. To top it all off, I developed something called GERD, which stands for gastro-esophageal reflux disease. I won't go into the details, but it meant that my stomach hurt—all the time. Some foods made it hurt worse.

Add the pain from GERD to the pain from the surgery and multiply that by the fact that I was dealing with the aftermath of the prostate biopsy—which is a whole other story—compounded by the unknown fear of the cancer itself and, well, you get the picture. Let's just say that the summer of 2011 was—with apologies to Mr. Dickens—the worst of times.

Let me interject something here about our youngest child, Jenna. We call her Boo Boo—but not for that reason. Jenna is the free spirit of the Huckaby clan. She is a thrill-seeker and her motor only runs at one speed and that is flat-out.

Jenna has given a lot of consideration to serving in the foreign mission field when she graduates from college. Lisa and I want her to be sure she knows what she is getting into so we have sent her on several mission trips.

She has been to Haiti a couple of times to help out earthquake victims and to New Orleans a couple of times to help out hurricane victims. She has made a couple of trips to Jamaica to work at a school for deaf children and has done inner city mission work in Indianapolis, although I warned her that she was wasting her time because those Yankees are beyond redemption.

We sent her to Kenya and to an Indian reservation in New Mexico and to Benin on the west coast of Africa for six weeks, where she traipsed through the jungles, from village to village, evangelizing to the people who are in the grips of voodoo and idol worship and black magic.

Everywhere we send Jenna, they keep sending her back.

In the summer of 2011 Jenna had answered the call of a program called Send Me Now. The program is sponsored by the Southern Baptist Missions Board and sends college students all over the globe. They sent Boo Boo to Glorieta, New Mexico, to work on the high adventure recreation staff at the LifeWay Christian Conference Center. That assignment was right up Jenna's alley. She spent twelve weeks running a zip line and a high ropes course, hiking through the Rocky Mountains and killing and cooking rattlesnakes. I knew I was in for a worrisome summer when after the first week of training she sent me an email telling me that her camp name was going to be "Danger."

Naturally we couldn't let our youngest child stay away from home for twelve weeks without visiting. So a couple of weeks after my surgery, we found ourselves on a plane, bound for Glorieta, about twenty miles west of Santa Fe. Actually, the plane was bound for Albuquerque. We were going to have to rent a car and drive to Santa Fe.

We spent eight days at the conference center and really had a great vacation. We got to meet Jenna's camp staff friends, including Smokey Lonesome, Tater, Moose, Rudy, Shadow, Grizzly—and a few others whose names I cannot recall. They were a great group of kids, and they seemed to enjoy having us hang out with them, especially when we drove and paid.

There were a couple of problems, however. I hurt the whole time we were there. I mean I really hurt. Plus I didn't have enough energy to punch my way out of a wet paper bag. I tried to be active and we walked around the campus and drove into Santa Fe several times and even went on a five-mile hike up the mountain. I don't recommend that two weeks after major surgery, by the way. The problem was, every time I spent half a day doing something, it took me a day and a half to recover. I spent a great portion of our vacation napping in the Hall of States, which is a very nice accommodation on the LifeWay campus.

The other problem was the G&G—GERD and gall bladder surgery. I could not tolerate eating meat very well and I could not tolerate eating spicy foods at all. You don't want to spend a week near Santa Fe, New Mexico, and not be able to tolerate spicy food. They put chili peppers in everything—and I mean everything. I ate two things the entire week that didn't cause excruciating pain. One was a Blizzard at the Dairy Queen in Pecos, a tiny town eight miles west of Glorieta on Route 66. The other was a hamburger at a quaint little adobe hole-in-the-wall called Bobcat Bite.

There is a funny story about Bobcat Bite. Jenna had known we were coming, of course, and had been on the lookout for a good place to eat with a lot of local flavor. She knows that we don't, as a rule, dine at chain restaurants when we are traveling. She had found the perfect place for us to try and we headed for it shortly after arriving in town.

Just as we were pulling into the parking lot of the dilapidated-looking building, my cell phone rang. I answered it and the voice on the other end said, "This is God calling. Where are you?"

I said, "If you are God, you ought to know where I am."

"You've got me there," admitted Marshall Edwards, the world's greatest Baptist preacher, who was on the other end of the call.

I advised him that we were visiting Jenna at Glorieta. After telling me how many times he had preached there and how great the snow skiing was in winter, he told me that I had to be sure to visit Bobcat

Bite for a hamburger. I laughed and told him that I was parked right in front of that historic establishment at that very moment and was going to indulge as soon as I got off the phone.

Now let me tell you about Marshall Edwards. I love him and I love his wife, Doris. Marshall and I both married way, way up, by the way.

Marshall moved to Newton County when he was a junior in high school and I was a small boy. His daddy and mine were friends, and I adored Marshall. Actually, the whole town did. He worked at White's, a department store on the Covington Square, and I wanted to be just like him when I grew up. I still do, come to think of it.

Marshall found Christ at a youth revival in 1957 at the Julia A. Porter Methodist Church and later went to Baylor University. It was a leap of faith because he did not have the money to pay for his education and did not know where the money was going to come from. But come it did. An anonymous benefactor paid his way through school. Every time he needed money to pay tuition or meet other needs, money arrived in his account, just like manna from heaven.

It wasn't until long after he graduated that Marshall learned that his benefactor had been Miss Mary Leila Ellington, his high school English teacher, who never had any children of her own. It was the best investment she ever made because Marshall became a preacher—and then some. He has preached of the love of Jesus Christ and His matchless grace on five continents, and has touched thousands and thousands of lives. I tell you this because it wasn't just a coincidence that Marshall called me at that precise time, as I would later learn.

I have to share one other story about our trip to New Mexico before I get back to the grim business of telling you about battling cancer. Jenna was working twelve- and sixteen-hour days while we were there, so we had to find ways to entertain ourselves most of the time. We spent a lot of time touring Santa Fe, which is an interesting town but very, very dry, and there was no place to swim at Glorieta. One day we went wading in a stream near Pecos, but we were dying to be submerged in water. At least I was. Lisa had had a tough spring, too, and was looking for a bit of pampering.

We found a little brochure in the lobby of the conference center touting a spa overlooking the city of Santa Fe called Land of 10,000 Waves. It bills itself as sort of a Japanese hot springs resort. One day we decided that we would take in the spa. Lisa called and made an appointment for a massage. I was looking forward to just relaxing by one of the pools.

Using our handy GPS, we arrived at the spa and it was very nice, with soothing music and a nice relaxing atmosphere. Lisa took the lead and checked in for her massage at the front desk. They gave her a cup of papaya juice—or something like that—and a robe and led her away to meet her masseuse.

I told the lady at the desk that I just wanted to use the sauna and steam room and hot tubs and the like. She gave me my robe and a cup of whatever Lisa was drinking and told me how to find my way to the amenities. As she handed me a towel she said that clothing was optional and that most people didn't wear bathing suits in the pools.

"Well, what do they wear?" I asked.

"Nothing," the attendant replied with a puzzled look.

Let me assure you, this old boy wasn't going to sit by the pool naked—or nude or nekkid, either. There is a great difference in being naked and being nekkid. As the late Lewis Grizzard so aptly put it, "Naked means you don't have any clothes on. Nekkid means you don't have any clothes on and are up to something."

I intended to be neither. I changed into my swimsuit in the men's room and found a lounge chair in an unobtrusive location in the corner of the spa room. As soon as I sat down, one of the most beautiful people I had ever seen, an Asian lady who looked to be about thirty, came out of the ladies' side of the dressing area, stood by the pool and dropped her kimono. All she had on was her birthday suit. I tried my best not to look, but honesty compels me to admit that my eyes did wander her way once or twice.

She did a series of stretching exercises and assumed a few yoga positions—she might have spent ten minutes on the pool deck—and then left. I am pretty sure she was an employee of the place and was sent there just to keep people's hopes up because everyone else who decided to sunbathe au naturel was like me and didn't have any business doing so.

After I had gotten over the shock of being at such an avant-garde facility, I went back to reading the book I had brought with me. It was Pat Conroy's "South of Broad," and I was reading it for the third time. I like all of Conroy's books but this one struck a particular nerve with me because it features a group of people who graduated from a Southern high school in 1970, the same year I did. These folks had to deal with integration and race relations and a lot of issues with which I was very familiar.

Anyway, as I was reading, two couples came out and got into the hot tub that was right in front of me. All four looked to be in their early seventies. Luckily they were fully clothed, like me.

They were very loud, especially one of the ladies, and I soon learned that they were from Chicago. The loud one in the bunch took note of my book and said, as if I weren't there, "That man is wasting his time reading that awful book about Charleston."

I peeked at her over the top of the book and she went on. "I read that book. It was terrible. And the author got Charleston all wrong. I know. I spent a weekend there."

One day I will learn to keep my mouth closed. It was not that day. I slowly lowered the book and in my silkiest Rhett Butler voice drawled, "Ma'am, realize that you are from Chicago and therefore know everything, but you must understand, Pat Conroy was raised in the South Carolina Low Country, graduated from the Citadel and spent a great deal of his adult life in Charleston—and he got it exactly right."

The lady didn't speak to me. She just looked around at her group and said, "Was he talking to me? Did that man say something to me?"

When her companions assured her that I had, indeed, spoken to her, she "harrumphed" and shook her head and exclaimed, "Well, I never!"

I looked her up and down and responded, "Yes, and you probably never will." Then I went back to devouring more of Conroy's splendid novel.

We had a grand time in New Mexico and it did provide us with a much-needed diversion, but it was soon time to return home and contemplate the tough decisions we had to make. Besides being very painful, my biopsy, you see, had provided us with some very sobering news.

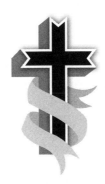

CHAPTER NINE

It is hard to describe the biopsy for prostate cancer, but I will try. Before I do, let me say this. If they would send a whole team of urologists to Guantanamo Bay next Monday and start giving daily prostate biopsies to the suspected terrorists—we'd know everything there is to know, including who killed Jimmy Hoffa, before the week was out.

First, there is the fear. Anytime you hear the "C-word," there is a fear of the unknown coupled with the fear that what you learn might be much worse than not knowing.

Having said that, the truth be known, I was more annoyed than I was afraid when I first learned that I might have cancer. I had heard all of the aforementioned lies about the disease. When Benny Potts, Lisa's dad, had prostate cancer, he underwent brachytherapy, or what most people refer to as "the seeds."

The way it works, as best I could figure out, is that a doctor surgically implants anywhere from fifty to one hundred radioactive seeds into the prostate gland, strategically placed based on the results of the biopsy. Then the patient goes for a specific number of daily radiation treatments. In Benny's case it was thirty. After that, problem solved.

I know dozens of men who have had and who are having this particular treatment, all with good results. Understand that this is not a medical journal and I am not a medical professional. My science may be a little off and I would never recommend any kind of treatment to any person. I am just telling my story.

YEA THOUGH I WALK

When I showed up at my local urologist on the Tuesday after my gall bladder surgery—before our trip to New Mexico—I was fully expecting to undergo the same treatments my father-in-law and others had undergone and was really irritated that I would have to stay around Conyers for a whole month just to get a ten-minute dose of radiation every day.

I am a busy man, don't you know—pause here for a snicker. I had places to go and people to see and things to do. I had a life to live. I had plans. And those plans did not include staying around home for a whole month during my summer off from school.

So that's how I showed up at the urologist. A little afraid, mostly from the stuff I read on the Internet, but above all, irritated and inconvenienced. Also I was hungry because I had to fast the day before. I don't want to be any more graphic than necessary, but I was getting very well acquainted with products produced by a certain Mr. C. B. Fleet of the Lynchburg, Virginia, Fleets.

My attitude would change in a hurry.

The doctor was very personable and very professional. He explained why we were there—"we" being Lisa and I—and tried to prepare me for what I would experience. No words could have prepared me for what I was about to experience. The nurse, who would soon become the doctor's partner in crime, was an old friend of Lisa's—who is a nurse herself, of course—and very familiar with us both. I am still not sure if that was a good thing or not.

When it got time for the biopsy, I had to take off my pants and get up on a table on my hands and knees. They sort of covered me up with one of those paper gowns, but y'all! It is impossible to maintain even a shred of dignity while hunkered down in such a position with one's wife, a nurse, and a doctor all in the room with you.

This is what they did. They placed an instrument filled with spring-loaded needles into my anus and all the way into the rectum. Apparently they have to put this apparatus a long way into the victim's—I mean, the patient's—interior and they had a hard time getting it far enough into mine. Lisa's friend kept telling me, "Relax. Relax, Darrell. Just relax."

Right. I wanted to tell her to swap places with me. I'd gladly have stood in the corner telling her to relax while she assumed the position.

Once the instrument—it's called a prostate gun, by the way—was sufficiently inserted, they started firing those needles, one at a time, into my prostate gland. I could hear the click of the gun before I felt the pain. The doctor told me it would sting a little. Bull feathers. It didn't sting a little. It hurt like the devil—and he did it over and over and over.

What I later learned was that, guided by a transrectal ultrasound probe, my physician was removing tiny little core samples from about a dozen places in my prostate gland. These cores would be tested for the presence of cancer cells. What I knew at the time was that it hurt like a son-of-a-gun every time he gathered one of his samples, and when it was all over, I was bleeding like a stuck pig—and would continue to bleed and to be sore as Lucifer for the next several days.

At first, I was confused when the doctor had told me that any surgery I might need couldn't take place until at least eight weeks after the biopsy. When I left his office that day, bloody and battered, I understood exactly why it would take my body at least two months to heal itself sufficiently to withstand surgery.

The week between having the operation and getting the results might have been the longest of my life, with the possible exception of the seven days leading up to the Sugar Bowl game between Georgia and Notre Dame following the 1980 football season. I wanted to go to that game, but I didn't have a car that would make the trip, had no money at all, and didn't have a ticket to the game. I could write a book about how I made my way to New Orleans that week.

Come to think of it, I already did. It is called "Need Two," and you can find out how to order it in the back of this book.

Of course, I made the mistake of trolling the Internet in the days following the biopsy. I played all the guessing games everyone plays, and my moods and my mind wandered all over the proverbial spectrum. There were times when I was convinced that my condition was terminal and I had only weeks to live. There were other times that I was absolutely certain that my cancer was fully contained and low grade. On those occasions I went back to being irritated that I would have to spend a month close to home.

Finally the moment of truth came. Lisa and I went back to my local urologist to get the results of the biopsy. That is the first time I heard the phrase that I would get so tired of hearing over the next twelve months. "Mr. Huckaby, I'm afraid it is a little worse than we thought."

Let me share a little about what I learned about prostate biopsies—other than how painful and humiliating they are. They are graded by something called the Gleason score, which measures the tumor patterns in the prostate. If you have a problem, your doctor can explain it more fully, but for general information, the possible Gleason scores range from 1 to 10, with 10 being the worst.

I got a 9. I also had cancer in both the left and right lobes of the prostate. It was also of a rare and very aggressive high-grade variety. I always have been an overachiever.

When the doctor gave us the verdict, I had no idea what all the mumbo jumbo meant. I felt a little proud of myself that I had achieved such a high number, in fact. I think my first response was to ask him something stupid like, "When can I get my seeds and start treatment."

That's when I started to understand, a little, what I was about to be facing. "I am afraid the seeds are not an option for you," he told me. "Your case is far too advanced and your type of cancer is far too aggressive. I strongly recommend a radical prostatectomy. In fact," he added, "I don't think you really have any other option."

I didn't like the term radical. I haven't trusted any radical since Thomas Jefferson and didn't enjoy hearing the term thrown around in conjunction with something somebody wanted to do to me. My heart sank when I heard this news and I am certain my face reflected my disposition.

The doctor began trying to reassure me. He explained what a prostatectomy would entail and all of the possible dangers and after effects. It turns out that a prostatectomy is one of the most intricate surgeries there is because the urethra runs right through the prostate, making it quite a trick to remove one while keeping the other intact and fully functional. No matter how skilled or how careful a surgeon might be, it is virtually impossible to perform this delicate surgery without affecting the nerves surrounding the urethra. This means that for most men, achieving and obtaining an erection will not be possible for many months.

Urinary incontinence, I was told, is the other major side effect, although it usually clears up a lot sooner than the erection issue. I know, too much information—but I want this story to be helpful as well as entertaining. It is what it is.

We were rocking along pretty well and I was trying to console myself to the fact that I would need surgery. The doc even told me that his partner, who he described as a "good old redneck boy," had been having a lot of luck with a comparatively new type of robotic surgery that is much less invasive, less likely to cause lasting nerve damage, and less debilitating. I could get back to my normal routine much faster if we opted for robotic surgery, in other words. Back to my normal routine sounded good to me because I do like normal and I do have a quite busy routine.

We were almost ready to pull the trigger and schedule the surgery, without even seeking a second opinion, when Lisa said something to my doctor about all my previous surgeries. She wanted to make sure the scars left behind would not create a problem.

The doctor seemed a bit taken aback by that and began asking questions about when the surgeries were and what they had entailed. I decided to make it easy for him. I stood and lifted my shirt to expose a stomach and chest crisscrossed with ugly red scars, many as wide as the doctor's thumb. I could read his mind. He wanted to ask about the knife fight and what the other guy looked like. When he saw that the newest and freshest scar ran far below my pants line, he just shook his head.

"I don't think you are a candidate for robotic surgery," he told me. "You have far too much scar tissue and probably lots and lots of adhesions. It would take too long and be too dangerous and I am not sure we could even do it."

Then he gave me the low-down on what "open surgery" might entail. Nothing on the menu sounded very delectable.

First of all, he couldn't schedule the surgery until late August and this was still early June. Remember when I said that I am not well acquainted with willpower? I have never even been introduced to patience. I didn't want surgery, but if I were going to have surgery, I wanted it immediately. I wanted the cancer out of my body and I wanted to begin the healing process so I could get on with my life.

When I relayed these wishes to the doctor, he said he understood, and then he reminded me of the painful biopsy and explained again that it would take time for the prostate to heal from that attack before he could safely remove it.

He explained what the operation would be like. He told me that I would probably have to stay in the hospital for about a week, wear a catheter for two or three weeks, and be laid up around the house and out of work—and circulation—for about eight weeks.

Eight weeks! That was an eternity! We weren't talking about doing the surgery until the end of August. I wouldn't be able to get out of the house until the end of October. I would miss the entire football season. What a depressing thought.

I just couldn't make a decision right then. I told my doctor that I would need some time to think about it. Again, he was very understanding and gave me a book that he said might help me reach a decision. It was called "The Decision," by John McHugh, a Gainesville urologist who had experienced prostate cancer himself. He opted for a radical prostatectomy and has recovered very well. His was an excellent book and it explained almost all of the medical options and described the pros and cons of each.

Dr. McHugh's book did, indeed, help me understand my options. Most of all he helped me understand that I did not want to undergo open surgery to have my prostate removed. Sadly, I thought that was the only option and had resigned myself to that option by the time we went back for the follow-up visit with our own urologist.

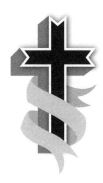

CHAPTER TEN

We pondered over the decision about surgery for about a week, I suppose. The doctor had said there wasn't a big hurry. I didn't understand his lack of urgency—or the lack of urgency of the entire medical system, to tell you the truth. I know. I know. I am not the first person to have cancer, and unfortunately, I won't be the last. The world didn't stop turning because I had cancer; there are more patients than healthcare professionals; I had to wait my turn; prostate tumors are usually slow-growing; and we had to wait for healing after the biopsy; and on and on and on ad nauseam.

I know all of that. I know every bit of that and I understand it. But it was me the cancer was growing inside of and it was urgent to me. I didn't want it taken care of in late August or even the next week. I wanted it to be taken care of last week. I wanted the cancer out of my body and I wanted to be on my way to healing.

I didn't want to be cut open, however. I had read Dr. McHugh's book thoroughly—some parts multiple times. I realized from what he said that my urologist was correct. The seed radiation didn't seem to be an option for me. The biggest drawback to the seeds seemed to be that if we tried the seeds and they didn't work—or if we tried them and the cancer came back—then surgery would not be an option. The only treatments available would be hormone therapy and chemotherapy, both of which have radical side effects and neither of which were seen as front-line remedies to my particular problem. There were places experimenting with proton therapy, which is a type of radiation that attacks only the cancer cells and carries less chance of damage to other organs and tissues, but with my high Gleason score, Dr. McHugh's information seemed to agree with my doctor's advice.

The prostate needed to be removed, taking the cancer with it.

Lisa set a follow-up appointment for me. To my dismay, when we arrived for the follow-up, my doctor was out of town and we met with a physician's assistant. I have nothing against PA's in theory, but this one didn't seem to have an ounce of familiarity with my case. He didn't seem to have glanced at my chart before walking in and sitting down. Every time we asked him a question, he seemed to be reading off a script. When we asked him questions specific to my case and my options, he stumbled around and didn't seem to quite have a handle on my unique situation. I am not trying to be harsh, but I left the facility depressed and upset and quite determined that I did not want to spend any more time with the PA.

In actuality, we had already resigned ourselves—again, "we" being Lisa and I, as this had been a team endeavor from the get-go. After further contemplation we decided to go ahead and meet with the urologist one more time and schedule the open surgery for the first available opportunity. August 28 became D-Day—and I became more depressed. I did not want to undergo an open surgery. It seemed too painful, the recovery seemed too long, and there seemed to be too much chance of permanent damage to too many functions that I had grown accustomed to. In short, I just lacked confidence in the whole process. A long summer became suddenly longer.

There is a funny thing about facing adversity. Some people claim that you can really find out who your friends are when the going gets tough and I would certainly agree. I suppose, conversely, you can find out who your friends aren't, too.

I had not shared my maladies with many people. Only my family members and a close circle of friends knew at that time, but word gets around in a small town. I suppose most people in the community knew that I had cancer, although they didn't know the extent of the illness. Most probably assumed as I had that prostate cancer wasn't too serious and that recovery would indeed be a piece of cake.

Our close Sunday school friends, the Hopes and the Walkers, were constantly looking in on me and feeding me and calling or texting. My buddy Gary, who is more a part of our family than not, became an even more permanent fixture than he had already been. My sister, Myron, whom I love with all my heart, probably wore out the buttons on her telephone calling to see how I was doing. Other friends with whom we were close became strangely absent from our lives.

I understand. Cancer makes some folks skittish. They don't know what to say or how to act and so they just keep their distance. I made up my mind during that period of time, however, that I would be much more vigilant in visiting my friends during times of need, even if I didn't really know what to do or say.

It was really kind of funny, though. When I would go out and about, a lot of people would tell me that they were "keeping up with me" through friends and relatives that I hadn't heard from in weeks or months. You gotta love people.

There was another serious problem I was dealing with all summer. The GERD. My stomach still hurt like fury, even after I got home from New Mexico and quit eating green chilies in every bite of food I was served. Our friend Carol Walker is one of the finest nurses I have ever known. She works for an internist and probably knows more about treating patients than most doctors have forgotten. She was instrumental in helping me find foods that I could easily digest and suggested I ask my own doctor for certain types of medicine that seemed to help some.

But here's the catch. There is always a catch, isn't there? While all this was going on, I was writing a cookbook. I ain't making this up. I was. "Second Helpings; The Southern Eatin' Cookbook."

You can't write a cookbook without trying out the recipes. At least I can't. All summer long, while Lisa was seeing patients and birthing babies, I was home cooking ribs and cornbread and fried chicken and all sorts of delectable dishes that Carol Walker was forbidding me to eat. The worst was when it was time to shoot the photographs of the food for the interior of the book and the cover. Every day for a couple of weeks I would cook enormous meals, arrange them just so on our kitchen table, take multiple photographs of the food, post them on Facebook, and then invite my friends and family over to eat what I had prepared while I sat glumly looking on.

Can you say pity party?

I still remember the day I shot the breakfast section. I had made bacon and sausage and the fluffiest scrambled eggs you've ever seen, and to top it all off, I had fried up several slabs of country ham and made red-eye gravy. The food looked so good spread out on the table that I just said to heck with it—did I mention the homemade biscuits?—and once I had finished taking the photographs, I ate everything in sight.

That was a year-and-a-half ago and my stomach still hasn't forgiven me.

My spirits and my attitude began to head toward rock bottom on the Fourth of July. We spent the day with Mark and Kathy Hope and a large number of mutual friends—plus all three of our children—at their Jackson Lake home. We had barbecue and fireworks and everyone swam and skied and a good time was had by all.

All, that is, except me. I was grateful to be included in the festivities and was happy to watch my kids tube and ski and laugh and play. But my stomach hurt and I couldn't eat and I couldn't ski, and the entire day I was wondering if this would be my last Independence Day celebration. I know. I was really a piece of work by this time.

Now you may be wondering at this point, "Why does he think I want to know all this?"

I realize that you may not, but there may be someone who is reading this book who is experiencing the same feelings I did and I want that person to know that they are not alone. Or maybe someone who has a friend or family member going through a similar ordeal will read these passages. I might help them understand how to help.

Or maybe you'll just learn what great Fourth of July parties Mark and Kathy Hope throw. At any rate, this is how I felt. But my main concern was that I was still unsettled about the choice I had made to have an open surgery. I kept reading more and more and more about the da Vinci robotic surgery system and I wanted so badly to have that as an option.

The day after the Fourth of July, I decided to seek an alternative path. I woke up that morning and did what I wish I had done weeks earlier. I called Carter Rogers.

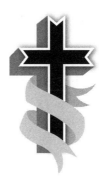

CHAPTER ELEVEN

Dr. Carter Rogers is a great American. He comes from a family of great Americans. His father, Bill, has been a pillar of the Conyers community for decades and is a proud native of the Palmetto State, as well as a Furman University graduate and former member of the United States Marine Corps. Carter's mother, Pat, is a retired school teacher and is also a proud Carolinian who traces her heritage all the way back to the American Revolution and before.

Carter's siblings are all outstanding in their own ways. One is a successful businesswoman and another is a pharmacist. Throw in an attorney and a Methodist preacher and you get the gist. Carter is good people and is from a family of good people.

What I like most about Carter is he is always the same, whether I see him uptown in his Bermuda shorts and an Augusta National polo shirt or at church, all dapper in his seersucker suit, bow tie and white bucks. He is down-to-earth, funny, and likes a good joke. Most of all, he cares about people, which is why he became a doctor.

Carter and I have a Salem Campground connection. Such can be said for many of my friends. His family has a "tent" just a couple of doors down from ours. I have known him since I married into the Cowan tent at Salem, about three decades ago.

Let's take another little detour here while I am talking about Dr. Rogers. When he was attending medical school at Georgia Regents University—sorry, Carter, and all other graduates of Medical College of Georgia—I wrote my first book, "Need Two." My publisher's wife was from Augusta and she set up my second-ever book signing at a chain store in Augusta. My first book signing had been in the friendly confines of a gift shop on the Covington Square. It was a smashing success, primarily because everyone in Newton County was anxious to find out if they were included in my novel. Most of them were, but I changed the names to protect the guilty.

Augusta was another kettle of fish altogether. I didn't know a soul in Augusta, and even though my agent assured me that there would be a lot of publicity in the Augusta paper about the event, I just knew that I would experience the humility of sitting a table all day, my face obscured by a tall stack of books that nobody wanted to buy.

That's the image I carried with me as I drove the two hours down Interstate 20 that Saturday morning. When I got to Augusta I almost kept going toward Myrtle Beach, but I decided to give it a shot and got off at the exit and headed to the bookstore. To my utter amazement there was a line waiting at my table when I arrived. It wasn't a wrapped-around-the-block line, but it was a this-will-take-a-while line, courtesy of the positive newspaper coverage, of course. The first person in line was my home boy, Carter Rogers. He has been one of my favorite people ever since.

One more Carter story. My mama was sick. Real sick. She was sick enough that we called in the nieces and nephews to say their goodbyes. She was hurting and in pain and just waiting to die. The doctors had done all that could be done. On the last full night my mother stayed on this earth, Carter was the surgeon on call. He didn't spend much time that night waiting for someone to operate upon. He spent most of that night in my mother's room, doing everything he could think of to ease her pain and make her comfortable.

I told you he was good people.

When I got Carter on the phone that day, I spilled my guts. I told him about all the pain I had been experiencing since October, about all the treatments, about the biopsy. I told him about my apprehensions about the surgery I was facing. I told it all. To his credit, never once did Carter say, "Dang, brother, I don't believe I'd told that."

He listened quietly until I had laid my entire burden right at his feet, metaphorically speaking. Then he set about trying to assuage my fears. He agreed with me that my urologist was a very good doctor and a very skilled surgeon. Given that, he told me that removing the prostate by open surgery was like "operating at the bottom of an orange juice can."

He didn't tell me that I should or should not pursue a second opinion or robotic surgery. What he did tell me was that he could put me in touch with other people who had experienced making that decision and that, if I chose to go that route, he could help me find someone who could do the surgery robotically, scar tissue and adhesions be damned.

I felt better immediately.

That evening I got a call as promised from Carter's friend, Dr. Brad Jacoby, in Covington, who knew first-hand the ordeal of having one's prostate removed long before he was ready to do without it. He was very helpful and helped ease a lot of my fears. I was scared to death of the catheter, for instance, but he convinced me that it wouldn't be as bad as I thought it would be. He lied, of course, but he still assuaged my fears.

We must have talked for an hour and I was becoming self-conscious about taking up so much of his time, but I also appreciated every minute of it because everything I heard from this survivor made me feel more comfortable about my situation. During the conversation, Brad laughed and said that his teenage daughter called him the "go-to guy" for men who had just been diagnosed with prostate cancer. That's a pretty good guy to be, I think.

Dr. Jacoby told me that one time he got really bored and went out to dinner while still wearing his catheter. I never did that, exactly, but I did make a speech to 600 while still wearing it. That's another story for another time. He also told me that his bell would still ring, although not as loudly or for as long as it once had. That was comforting news indeed. He gave me the name and number of his physician and offered to help me get an appointment if I needed one.

Later that week, Wales Barksdale, a longtime friend, gave me a call. Wales is also from a prominent Conyers family and chairman of our county school board. He buys his drugs—excuse me, his pharmaceuticals—from my daughter and had kept up with my condition through her. He also gave me the name of a good friend, Bill Archer, who had walked my path. I had a long conversation with Bill, who is a member of the University of Georgia Athletic Board, and he mentioned the name of the same surgeon Brad Jacoby had mentioned. I decided to give Scott Miller a call. I think it was one of the best decisions I have ever made.

You might notice a couple of things if you have been following closely. For the first month or six weeks of my having been diagnosed with prostate cancer, I tried to figure everything out for myself. I never really asked for too much help—from anyone I knew or from God. That didn't work out very well. I am a pretty tough guy and have always been a competitor, but I learned that I wasn't big enough to fight cancer alone.

As soon as I turned to others for help, I started feeling better about my predicament. As soon as I turned the entire matter over to God, I would find peace. Peace would be a long time in coming, but I was about to take the first step in that direction.

Remember the God-instances I mentioned earlier. I was about to experience another.

I called Dr. Scott Miller's office and got an appointment for a consultation at one o'clock on the afternoon of July 15, which happened to be my lovely wife, Lisa's, fiftieth birthday. The day after I made that call marked the first day of Salem Camp Meeting, and for the next eight days I would be engulfed and uplifted by the sweet, sweet spirit that is in that place.

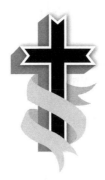

CHAPTER TWELVE

The first camp meeting in the United States was held in 1801 in Cane Ridge, Kentucky. Twenty-three years later, a group gathered for two weeks near a spring on what is now Salem Road in Covington, Georgia, and a tradition was established that has lasted for almost 200 years.

Salem Camp Meeting is a lot of things to a lot of people. It is part ritual, part family reunion, part vacation—but most of all, it is a revival meeting; a chance to get closer to God, to examine one's soul, to refresh one's spirit. If anyone ever needed one's soul examined or one's spirit refreshed, it was I when everyone began to gather under the outdoor tabernacle on the eighth day of July in the year of our Lord, 2011, to sing "Sweet, Sweet Spirit," the annual theme song at Salem.

I accepted Christ at a very young age. I should have known from the very beginning that I couldn't fight cancer by myself. I did know, and yet I tried to do it anyway. I should have turned the whole burden over to the Lord when I first was diagnosed. St. Paul wrote in his letter to the early church at Philippi, "Do not be anxious about anything, but in every situation, by prayer and petition, with thanksgiving, present your requests to God." Philippians 4:6 (NIV)

Don't hear something I am not saying. I had prayed throughout my illness. I have prayed just about every day of my life—ever since my mama used to tuck me in and listen to my "Now I lay me down to sleep" petitions every night. There is a difference, however, in praying about something and turning something completely over to God. I can't say that I reached that point during camp meeting that summer, but I can say that I got a lot more in tune with God during the week.

It was a strange week. Just about everyone on the campus knew that I had cancer, but I hadn't really talked openly about it to many people. I was still trying my best to keep it inside. I still hoped against hope that the surgery would fix everything and that after I was healed and back to my old self I could brag about beating the Big C.

Because I hadn't talked to many people about it, not many people would mention it to me. I would pass people on the grounds and they would try to avoid making eye contact. They would nervously mumble something like, "I've been thinking about you," and hurry on their way. I was just as evasive as they were, and maybe more so.

To make matters worse, I was still struggling with the aftermath of my other surgeries and was still battling the strange pain in my stomach and chest. I didn't have a very pleasant week, understand. As soon as evening worship services ended, I would go back to our tent and sequester myself in my room. Normally at Salem, I would sit on the front porch until midnight, solving the problems of the world with Daniel Farley and Joe Cook and Ken Parkinson, or talking football and politics with Nat Long. Not this year.

I couldn't fall asleep in my room. I would just lie there in the bed until Howard Kennedy, the camp bugler, played "Taps" and the campground went dark. When Lisa came to bed, I would go and stretch out on the front porch swing so that my tossing and turning wouldn't bother her. More than once that week, I was still on the front porch swing when Howard played reveille the next morning.

There were a few people I did talk with about my illness that week. One was our friend Diane Howington—the lady with whom, you'll recall, I "had my first child".

When her firstborn, Marci, was a toddler, Diane was running Gailey's Shoes and had to go to work every day. Lisa was working, too, at the hospital. I was the babysitter during the Salem Camp

Meeting. Diane would drop off Marci at our back door every morning, and she and Jamie Leigh would spend the day together, going to classes, doing crafts, playing at the spring, and doing all the things toddlers do at Salem.

A couple of years later, we were delighted when Diane decided to take over her family's cabin, the Plunkett tent, and started staying the week on the campground. She has been a fixture ever since, and her front porch is like an oasis for all of us who are thirsting for relief from the pressures of our own close quarters.

You see, at Salem, several families usually cram themselves into one small cabin—what we call "tents"—for the week. It's pretty easy to get on one another's nerves in such a setting. Diane, however, maintains a laissez faire atmosphere around her tent that the rest of us tenters envy. When the going gets tough—or when I need to sneak an unhealthy snack—I go to Diane's front porch. I spent a lot of time on her front porch that week.

Sometimes we sat and talked. Sometimes we sat and laughed. Sometimes we sat and cried. Sometimes we just sat.

Another person I spent a lot of time with that week was Bishop Bubba. Actually, his name is really Hugh Hendrickson. Hugh became a regular at Salem during his teen years and is a regular on Diane's front porch. He was known for most of his life as Bubba, but since becoming an ordained Methodist elder, he has tried to live that down and be recognized by his more scholarly given name. Sometimes we remember and sometimes we don't, thus the moniker, "Bishop."

Above all else, Bubba is a caring, genuine person and is good at listening. He listened to me a lot during camp meeting that year.

Our days are pretty full at Salem. We have morning watch at 7:30 a.m. each day. The messages at morning watch used to be short devotionals that have evolved into a series of mini-sermons over time. We have hour-long Bible studies at 9:30, followed by morning worship, which consists of gospel singing and a sermon, and then everyone retreats to their respective tents for lunch. Some folks stay in the Salem Hotel that is in a prominent corner of the campground. They take their meals there.

The afternoon is reserved for porch sitting and visiting. Suppers are enormous smorgasbords of traditional Southern dishes, at least at our tent and the hotel dining room. The main worship service of the day begins at 7:45 p.m. and lets out around 9:15 p.m. That's when we head back to the tent to spend an hour or so fellowshipping with a couple of dozen of our closest friends and eating homemade ice cream.

Yes, we have homemade ice cream every night—usually two kinds: peach and another flavor.

The point to all this is that during the eight days of camp meeting, a person battling cancer, or any other demon, has a lot of time to think and to give God a chance to help carry the load. I finally began to do that as the week wore on.

It just so happened that I was asked to give the devotional at morning watch on the last Friday of the week. It was a big day. It was Lisa's fiftieth birthday, for one thing, and it was the day that I would finally get to see Dr. Scott Miller, for another.

I had been planning my mini-sermon for a while and wanted to talk about Tony Fontaine, a Hollywood actor and magnificent singer who was very popular nationwide in the 1960s. He was also an evangelist and preached at Salem one year. He died just a few months later, but I had never known the cause. As I was researching his life for my sermon notes, I learned that he died of prostate cancer, just a few months after having been diagnosed.

I was shocked to learn that and shared it with those gathered under the tabernacle that Friday morning. As I was relating this, I looked out into the congregation and saw my friend Bishop Bubba wiping a tear from his cheek.

Things were going to get better that day, however. I had an appointment with the robotics guy at one o'clock. I had never been so glad to have an appointment with a doctor.

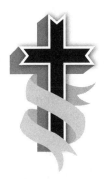

CHAPTER THIRTEEN

I have never heard anyone brag, "I went to the seventh best doctor in Atlanta," or "I have the twelfth best surgeon in the Southeast." Everybody always wants the best doctor available and I am no exception.

I want to make one thing perfectly clear. I appreciate and respect every medical professional who has treated me over the past two years—or ever for that matter. The fact that I chose to seek out a consultation has nothing to do with my local doctor—except that he said his group could not do my surgery because of the complications caused by my previous surgeries. Who knows? I might have been better off having the open surgery. We'll never know, but if I had it to do over again, I would follow exactly the same path I followed—except for one thing.

If I had it to do it over, I would have followed the sage advice of my friend Wayne Kinnett, who is himself a survivor of prostate cancer. When I was diagnosed and called him for advice he said, "My first advice would be not to get prostate cancer."

I wish I had called Wayne earlier.

Once I knew that surgery was inevitable, I started investigating all the possibilities and side effects and after effects of the various treatments available, and the more I read, the more convinced I became that my best option was robotic surgery using the da Vinci surgical system, a technological marvel that allows surgeons to perform minimally invasive procedures for complex medical conditions. The da Vinci is used for all sorts of surgeries but seems to have been invented for the removal of the prostate gland. And, no, I am not a paid spokesperson—but maybe I should be.

The more I read about the da Vinci, the more convinced I was that I wanted that type surgery, and when I read about the da Vinci, one name kept coming up, over and over and over—Dr. Scott Miller. As we drove away from Salem that Friday morning and headed up I-20 toward Northside Medical Center in Atlanta, where Dr. Miller's offices are housed, my fervent prayer had become that he would tell me he could perform my surgery.

I don't know what I expected when I got to Dr. Miller's office, but it was nothing like what actually happened. We navigated the parking decks and the maze of office buildings at Northside and found the combination of elevators and hallways that would take us to the outer office of Georgia Urology, with whom Dr. Miller is associated.

It is always a bit sad to sit in a doctor's waiting room, knowing that everyone there has a serious medical condition. I always find myself scanning the faces of the people, wondering what is wrong with each person and how they are coping, all the while knowing that they are wondering the same thing about me.

We got to the office well before our appointment time—my pet peeve in life is tardiness. I had thumbed through every magazine in the office that had pictures of football players or pretty girls and had started the second round when we were called into Dr. Miller's inner waiting room. Here I met Valerie for the first time. Valerie is Dr. Miller's nurse and would become my very best friend in the whole world about six weeks later when she removed my catheter, one week after my surgery. On this day, however, she was simply the nice nurse who took my health history and offered me a Coca-Cola while I waited.

I had never been offered a Coke in a doctor's office before. I thought that was pretty cool.

Honesty compels me to admit that we waited awhile before we were called back to actually talk to the doctor, but we soon learned why. He was in no hurry whatsoever. He treated us like we were the only two people in the whole world once we got back into his plush office.

I liked Scott Miller immediately. He was wearing a shirt and tie, not a lab coat or scrubs. We were offered seats in two very comfortable chairs. Dr. Miller sat and faced us. He crossed his legs casually and began to engage us in conversation. We talked to him about our jobs and our children and where we were raised and educated. Then we talked about his background and his children and their educational experiences. He was very interested in my teaching methods and prescriptions for helping his daughter succeed in her AP classes during the coming school year.

I was reminded of Lee's meeting with Grant at Appomattox. According to history, General Lee arrived at the meeting with Grant attired in full dress uniform. Grant came in all muddy and grimy in his field blues. Dr. Miller would have been Lee for the sake of this comparison. But Lee was eager to talk about the business at hand while Grant wanted to reminisce about the Mexican War and old times not forgotten. I was like General Lee in this regard. I just wanted to know if the doc could take out my prostate and he acted like that was the last thing on his mind.

Lisa and I fully enjoyed the conversation but I finally just asked him point blank about the chances of him doing the surgery. He glanced through my charts, with which he was already familiar, and said, "Certainly I can do it. Are you sure that's what you want?"

I must have sounded pretty stupid when I asked if he wanted to see my scars. He just looked a bit bemused and said, "Not really. I'm sure I can deal with them."

I pulled up my shirt and made him look at my stomach anyway.

He assured me once again that he could handle the surgery robotically. Then he started going over the after effects of the surgery, just so we would both know what we were getting into.

"You will not be able to perform sexually for about eight months after the surgery," he told me.

"Oh, I don't perform now," I told him. "We do all that stuff in private."

He looked at me like I was a bit odd and said, "No, you don't understand. You won't be able to have sex for about eight months."

At this point Lisa spoke up and said, "We'll pay double if you can make it twenty months."

I was in a bidding war with my own wife and she makes a lot more money than me.

Scott Miller has probably removed thousands of men's prostate glands but he has never had a patient more relieved than I was when he told me he could do my surgery. He explained exactly how he would do it and exactly what the recovery would be like and then we walked back to get my surgery on the calendar.

August 10 would be the day. It was a Wednesday, right in the middle of the week. It would be done robotically, which was a load off my mind. I had infinite confidence in my doctor, in great part because he had great confidence in himself. And we were doing it two weeks earlier than we could have done the open surgery. That was good, too. Two weeks sooner until full recovery.

Life was good when we left the tall office tower at Northside and headed back to Salem for the last night of camp meeting—and I would sleep better that night than I had in months.

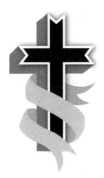

CHAPTER FOURTEEN

I was a little more upbeat after meeting with Dr. Miller and finally knowing exactly what path we were about to follow to deal with this nasty disease. I was confident that the surgery would work and I began to think about writing my funny little guide about dealing with prostate cancer. I would call it, as I said, You Took Out My What?!

There were a few things to take care of prior to surgery, however. Like school. I was about to enter my thirty-eighth year as a classroom teacher and I was absolutely certain that Heritage High School, where I had taught AP U.S. History for the past fourteen years, could not function without me. If they could, I didn't want them to find that out.

God was smiling on that situation. The previous year a remarkable young man named Patrick Kicklighter had spent a semester doing his student teaching at Heritage. He was willing to be my long-term substitute and, supported by the magnificent Hanahans—Peggy and her son, Marion, both of the Alabama Capstone—I knew my classes would be in good hands.

I tried my best to convince myself that everything was fine and that the surgery and recovery would be a piece of cake. I promised myself that I wouldn't worry about anything, that I would shake off the surgery after a few days, and that I would be back to normal in a matter of weeks.

The problem was, I was lying to myself. I hadn't even been able to shake off the surgery I had in June. I had very little energy and was still dealing with that mysterious stomach pain that no medication, diet, or treatment had seemed to ease.

YEA THOUGH I WALK

I was scared and depressed and, late at night, in the privacy of my bedroom, I would lie awake and talk to God about my problems without ever giving God a chance to talk back. I never listened for that still, quiet voice that would give me blessed assurance that things would be OK. I simply told God what I was going to do and what I needed instead of leaning on Him and asking for guidance.

I was determined that I would be master of my own fate. He who is master of his own fate serves a fool. You may quote me on that.

As my surgery grew closer and closer, I became more and more of a hot mess. I have always bragged that I wasn't afraid of anybody or anything—and for the most part, that claim was not filled with false bravado. But as July was about to turn into August in 2011, I was scared, although I would never have admitted it. I was pretending to be brave and invincible and was trying to carry a heavy, heavy load all by myself.

On the last Saturday in July, I would encounter another of those providential God-instances that I have become so cognizant of over the past year or so. I was invited to the Georgia Club in Statham to play in the Georgia Club Foundation's annual celebrity golf tournament, even though I am neither a golfer nor a celebrity.

Frank Chandley and his wife, Katherine, live at the Georgia Club and are a part of the Oak Tree Gang tailgate group. Their group graciously invited Lisa and me to join them for tailgating under the oak trees on Agriculture Drive before Georgia home football games. Apparently a lot of the good people who live at Georgia Club read my weekly column in the Athens Banner-Herald and asked Frank to invite me to their charity tournament.

I'm not one to turn down an invitation, especially when that invitation affords me the opportunity to eat two good meals, hang out with Bulldog greats like George Patton, Andy Johnson, and Ray Goff, and media greats like Chuck Dowdle and David Chandley, Frank's son and my favorite television weather guy.

I told you all of that to tell you this. I wasn't even able to pretend to play golf at this particular outing, so I was allowed to ride around the course in a golf cart driven by my friend, Buddy Neel. Buddy lives at the Georgia Club too, and is quite an interesting fellow, despite being a Florida Gator. He has lived and worked all over the country and the world and has a great insight into the human condition.

We enjoy riding together because we can share the problems of the world between golf shots.

The extent of my physical activity on the particular day was to putt the ball on each green so the real players could evaluate the speed of the greens and see how their own putts might break. I got lucky and sank a couple of long ones, so that was pretty cool.

Mostly, I just sat in the cart, as I said, and talked to Buddy.

We were about halfway around the course when Buddy said, out of the blue, "I heard you are fighting cancer."

I was a bit surprised that Buddy was aware, but simply answered, "Yes, I am."

Buddy responded in a matter-of-fact manner that was direct and to the point. "Why haven't I read about it in your column?"

That really took me aback. "I don't know," I mumbled. "It's just sort of private and not something I would really share with my readers."

"Well you should," was his reply.

"Why?" I asked.

"Because you could help a lot of people. There are lots of guys and their families going through what you are. You could be an encouragement to them. Besides," he continued. "There are a lot of people who would like to support you and pray for you."

Then Buddy Neel nodded toward a large boulder on the edge of the course. "What if you had to carry that big rock?" he asked. "Would you try to lift it by yourself or would you ask folks to help you?"

"I'd ask for help," I admitted. "That thing is heavy."

"Is it heavier than trying to battle cancer by yourself?" Buddy asked. "The more people carrying a load, the lighter that load becomes. There are thousands of people who would be willing to help you carry your load. You need to give them a chance."

That was that and we went back to talking about the upcoming football season and the price of tea in China—where Buddy had worked for a number of years.

I gave his words a lot of thought throughout the following week. That weekend I decided that I would heed his advice and I spilled my heart in the next Sunday's column.

A couple of things happened. First of all, my email inbox began to light up like a pinball machine. There were letters of support and promises of prayers from all over Georgia and beyond the state's borders—and those messages would continue to come for weeks. One of my friends sent me a message that I really should log on to the online version of my column and read the messages of goodwill that had been left for me. This person knew that I wasn't in the habit of reading the online comments to my columns because so many people are so critical.

I followed his advice, though, and was amazed at the hundreds of people who wanted to wish me well—even some of my harshest critics, like Athens legend Ed Tant, had words of hope and encouragement. It was really an uplifting experience.

Two days later, letters and cards started flooding my mailbox. The U.S. Postal Service got a major lift the first week of August and the cards and letters kept coming throughout the fall—by the thousands.

I had never felt more affirmed and more encouraged in my entire life, and I cherished each and every comment, phone call, email, letter, and Facebook post. All of those things were quite tangible and concrete, but there was something supernatural going on, too. I began to experience a feeling of peace about my situation that I had not known since my diagnosis had been made. I could fall asleep at night. I slept through the night. I was experiencing a lot less trepidation and fear.

Finally I realized the source of my newly found peace. I was experiencing first-hand the amazing supernatural power of intercessory prayer. I realized that because I had taken Buddy Neel's advice and given my friends and fans and total strangers the opportunity to lift my name to the Lord, because I had allowed others to share my load, that load was becoming lighter and lighter.

The thing was, I already knew that is what would happen. I just needed a gentle nudge in the ribs to remind me. Instead, I got a swift kick in the pants—and one for which I will be forever grateful.

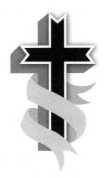

CHAPTER FIFTEEN

It is amazing how medical care—especially surgery—has changed over a generation. When I was twelve, my father had cataract surgery at what was then called Georgia Baptist Hospital. He was there for a week, at least, and my mother stayed with him most of the time. My cousin, Buck Bouchillon, drove me to Atlanta to see him a couple of times.

My daddy was a scary sight, sitting up in bed in his pajamas with his head immobilized lest a certain movement might tear out his stitches. He had a stubble of a white beard and a white bandage over half his face. The visits made quite an impression on me because I can still remember them in great detail. I can also remember Buck taking me over near Georgia Tech following those visits to have supper at Lester Maddox's Pickrick Restaurant.

The year 1964 was turbulent in the American South. Following passage of the 1964 Civil Rights Act, previously all-white restaurants began to serve customers of all races. Not Lester Maddox, though. He claimed that his private property rights were being violated and vowed to fight the federal agents and outside agitators who threatened to integrate his establishment, by force if necessary.

During my daddy's stay at Georgia Baptist, Lester's restaurant was being picketed—he insisted that the protestors were "outside agitators"—and I think Buck, who was a political junkie like me, enjoyed all the drama and appreciated the historic perspective. I was twelve. All I knew was that Lester and Virginia Maddox served some really good fried chicken.

I can still see him in my mind's eye walking around his place of business, bald head gleaming, holding a pot of coffee in one hand and a pitcher of sweet tea in the other, chatting with visitors and refilling cups and glasses. I can also still see in my mind's eye the gun rack on the wall filled with a dozen pick handles.

My visit to Northside Hospital was nothing like my daddy's stay at Georgia Baptist. If there was any political unrest in the area, I was unaware.

I woke up early on the day of my surgery. It felt like game days used to feel when I coached high school football and basketball. Uplifted by the thousands of prayers that been sent heavenward on my behalf, I was at peace with what was about to happen and had full confidence in Scott Miller's abilities to do what needed to be done.

We navigated the Interstate 285 rush hour traffic and arrived at Northside well ahead of time. The check-in process was a breeze. They took me back to a holding cell—at least that's what it felt like to me—and Dr. Miller came in to say hello and give me one more chance to back out. I'm kidding about the last part. It felt funny to see Dr. Miller in his green scrubs and a do-rag. I had only seen him in dress clothes. He told us we were second on the runway and wished me luck.

The day went downhill from there.

I don't like waiting. Somehow the patience gene passed me by completely. When I coached basketball, I always hated it when the preliminary game went into overtime. When I got myself psyched up and ready, I was ready.

That day I felt like the astronauts must have felt—back when America still had a manned space program—when the countdown clock got stuck at T-minus twenty minutes and holding. The nurses came in and dressed me in a gown, put an IV in my arm, and gave me a little something to help me relax. I was good to go—only we didn't get to go. An emergency case came in before us or something happened. I'm not sure what. What I do know is that I became very agitated and probably didn't behave very well.

Lisa told me that a crowd had gathered in the waiting room—I think the preacher was out there along with some of our close friends and people from our Sunday school class. Cousin Kristina was there—Kris is always there for us. Jamie and Jackson, our two older children, were in attendance. Jenna—aka, Danger—was still fighting the good fight at Glorieta—and, of course, my sister, Myron, was there.

Let me tell you about my sister. She is one of the best people God ever placed on this earth and is certainly one of the sweetest. I think John F. Kennedy was president when she and her husband, Steve Singley, started dating. Steve is a great guy, too, and was voted best looking freshman at Newton County High School two or three years in a row.

In 1966, when I was in the ninth grade and Myron was a senior, Steve received notice that his Uncle Sam required his services in the armed forces of the United States. Shortly after he completed his basic training at Fort Benning, Georgia, and further artillery instruction at Fort Sill, Oklahoma, Steve was given a few days off to come home and tell everyone goodbye before leaving for a year-long all-expense-paid trip to Southeast Asia. More specifically, he was being sent to Vietnam.

I was clueless, of course. I was fourteen and in love with life. I was two or three weeks into high school and had been introduced to a whole new world at our county's consolidated high school. I had been in classes with kids from Porterdale—kids just like me, whom I had known all my life—for the first eight years of my public education. Newton High, on the other hand, was full of new and interesting people—not to mention beautiful girls that I had never met.

It was a Friday night in September. Gone With the Wind was playing at the Strand Theater on the Square in Covington. I had read GWTW for the first time when I was in the fourth grade. My cousin Carolyn had given me a copy. I had read it a half-dozen times since and had seen the movie so many times that I knew every line by heart. But I had never watched it with anyone as pretty as Karen Meadors, and on this particular Friday night I had somehow convinced her to meet me at the Strand and sit with me during the show. Did I mention that Gone With the Wind is four hours long? Just a little slice of heaven!

By the time Scarlett made her first big mistake and married Charles Hamilton, we were sitting really close together. By the time Scarlett danced with Rhett Butler at the bazaar, I was holding her hand. I am pretty sure I had never held a girl's hand before, at least not in public. I had never had such a feeling.

Suddenly, a bright light was shining right in my eyes. "Here he is, Mrs. Huckaby! He's with a girl, too!"

The lisping voice was that of long-time Strand usher, Foy Harper. My mother had come into the theater and told Foy that I just had to be found. Never let it be said that Foy Harper would shirk his duty during critical times.

I was shocked that my mama was looking for me in the theater and mortified that she and Foy broke up my promising evening. I mumbled my goodbyes and hurried with Foy to the lobby.

This is what was happening. Steve was shipping out for 'Nam on Monday. He and Myron, who was 17 at the time, decided that neither could survive his deployment if they weren't married. Georgia had a waiting period to get married. South Carolina did not. Myron, Steve, my parents, along with Steve's parents and his sister and brother-in-law were all headed to the nearest border to witness the nuptials.

I was outraged that I had to leave the theater for something as trivial as a wedding ceremony. My outrage and a quarter would have gotten me a bag of popcorn and a small Coke at the Strand concession stand but it didn't get me anywhere with Tommie Huckaby. I didn't have to go to South Carolina, primarily because there wasn't room for me in the car. I did have to go home, however, so my mother wouldn't have worry about where I was all night.

Who knows how my life might have turned out if Karen Meadors and I had been allowed to make it to the scene where Scarlett shot the Yankee intruder or the one where Rhett carried her upstairs and kicked the bedroom door open? Certainly not me, but what I do know is that Steve and Myron are still married and that there has never been a crisis in my life, real or imagined, that my sister wasn't right there to give me her support.

The day of my prostatectomy would be no different, of course. She wanted to come back and visit me where I was waiting. Everybody wanted to come back and visit. But I didn't really want to see anybody. I was in a backless gown and was hooked up to all sorts of machines and needed to get up and go pee every ten minutes. To make matters worse, Dr. Miller was delayed so long that the little something they had given me to calm my nerves wore off and the peace I had known when I arrived at the hospital was all but gone.

I still let my sister come back to see me, of course. Who can say no to someone who loves him so unconditionally? Besides, the feeling is mutual.

Finally God sent a beautiful blue-eyed angel to my rescue. Actually, I made that up. It was a nurse, I think, not an angel, and she could have been as ugly as Miss Boo for all I knew or cared. Someone finally came in, however, and told Lisa to give me a kiss. Then the nurse—or whoever it was—gave me one of those magical injections that sends you off to la-la land. I was asleep before they rolled the stretcher down the hall.

I don't know what happened between, say, noon on that Wednesday in August and 8 o'clock that night. Something tells me I don't want to know. I have been told that our good friend Mark Hope, who has fought beside me every inch of the way in this battle, took everybody in the lobby along with one or two strangers over to Perimeter Mall to dine at Maggiano's Little Italy, a wonderful restaurant where enormous bowls of succulent Italian food are served family style, along with fresh salad and hot bread. I was upside down on an operating table for five hours and they were living it up at Maggiano's— and I am eternally thankful to Mark that they were. Of course, he did promise me later that he would take me as soon as I was able to enjoy it. I think the time is about ripe.

They tell me that because Dr. Miller had to use such precision and care cutting through all the adhesions and scar tissue in my abdomen that the operation, which was expected to last a couple of hours, instead lasted more than four hours, and closer to five. Luckily, Dr. Miller doesn't get time-and-a-half for overtime.

YEA THOUGH I WALK

I couldn't see myself when I came out of surgery, which is a good thing. I was told later that because I was suspended upside down for so long, my face had filled with blood and had become bruised and swollen. I looked, so they say, like a person from another planet. I always knew I was out of this world.

When I came to, I wished I were in another world. I hurt, which was to be expected, but worse than the pain was the feeling that I had to urinate. I didn't, of course, because the doctor had inserted the dreaded Foley catheter during surgery, but the urge was there and it was one of the worse feelings I have ever experienced. I kept telling Lisa and the nurse and anyone else who would listen that I had to go—and they kept telling me that I didn't. This went on for a couple of days. It could have been much worse. I have since talked with other unfortunate souls who experienced these bladder spasms for weeks.

This is very rare, however, so if you need a prostatectomy, don't let the possibility of bladder spasms scare you away. If I can survive them, you can, too.

I don't remember much about the long night in the hospital following surgery. I do recall that a nurse came in at about 2 a.m. and was horrified to realize that I hadn't been made to walk yet. She got me out of bed and she and I walked down the hall and back. She bragged on me so much that I felt like I had won an Olympic marathon. The rest of the night is a blur. I whined and cried and begged for pain medicine and kept insisting that I needed to pee.

They gave me pain medicine when they could, and my new trainer had me walking around and around the whole wing by morning. I think I ate something around breakfast time. I kept begging to go home, in between begging for pain medicine and screaming that I needed to pee. That was pretty much my day. I remember being told that I couldn't go home until I had experienced the all-important bowel movement. That magic moment occurred around 4:30 in the afternoon, and at 5:00 I was wheeled down to the front lobby while Lisa brought the car around. We were set free, right into rush hour traffic—in the middle of a torrential rainstorm.

C'est la vie!

The first evening at home was not intolerable. I hurt, of course, and I almost passed out when I lifted my shirt and looked in a mirror. I had seven incisions of varying depths and lengths all over my lower abdomen. Those perfectly complemented the other large scars across my chest. I looked like I had somehow survived a sword fight with Zorro—but just barely. I made everybody who came to see me for the next month look at my scars and I couldn't wait to go to the beach and take off my shirt.

The catheter was a nuisance that first night and would become much more than a nuisance before the week was out. All in all, however, I was glad to be home and in the relative comfort of my own recliner.

Day two at home, however, would be exponentially worse.

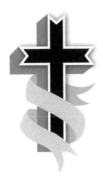

CHAPTER SIXTEEN

In the immortal words of the late Larry Munson, "Alright now, get the picture!"

I woke up on Friday morning after my radical prostatectomy on Wednesday. Come to think of it, how could there be a prostatectomy that wasn't radical? There were seven incisions in my abdomen and each of them felt like the scalpel, or whatever torture device the da Vinci uses to make incisions, was still in place. There was a thick plastic tube running out of my penis—I am sorry, there is no polite way to say it—and into a urine collection bag hooked to the side of my bedstead. My most minute movement caused the catheter to pull and it hurt like fury. When I didn't move, it was merely uncomfortable.

Now assume that every portal in the body is sealed up—I'm talking mouth, ears, rear-end, everything—and someone keeps pumping gas into that sealed up body as if it were a helium balloon that would not give, much less break. That's the way I felt on my second day at home. It might have been the most miserable day I have ever spent.

I moaned. I groaned. I ranted. I raved. I whined. I cried. I prayed for someone to shoot me and put me out of my misery.

My lovely wife, Lisa, who has been a Registered Nurse and a Registered Nurse Midwife for thirty years and is immune to pain—as long as it is someone else's—showed me little sympathy. OK. That was a lie. She showed me no sympathy. In fact, I think she was enjoying my misery. She probably saw it as payback for the three times she went through labor with our children.

"Get on your hands and knees," she told me. "That will help the gas move around."

"Where did the gas come from?" I demanded. "I haven't eaten anything but Jell-O for three days!"

"The doctor used gas to inflate your stomach," she explained for the umpteenth time, "so he could see to perform the surgery easier."

"Ooooooh!" was the only reply I could make.

"Lie on your left side," she suggested. "That's what we tell pregnant women when they have gas pains."

I wished I were pregnant. If I had been, I would have been pretty certain that the pain would ease after nine months. I was convinced that the gas pains I was experiencing were permanent.

"Get up and walk around," was Lisa's next solution.

I tried. I really did try. Every time I stood up I seemed to step on the catheter tube. Every time. The only thing worse than having a tube sticking out of the end of your penis is for that tube to be yanked on ten or twelve times a day.

I sat—or crawled on my hands and knees—watching the clock all day, praying for nightfall and my next sleeping pill. I felt like I was living through the day described in Joshua 10:13. "The sun stopped in the middle of the sky and delayed going down a full day."

That was the only day during this entire ordeal that I got really angry with Lisa. It wasn't about something she did, it was about something she didn't do—something I had begged her to do for weeks before the surgery.

My buddy, Wayne Kinnett, the one who advised me not to get prostate cancer to begin with, gave me one other piece of advice a couple of days before my surgery. He told me to be sure and pick up one of those elevated toilet seats. He was convinced that the makers of the standard toilet and the makers of the standard catheter tubes were in cahoots. No matter what you do, you cannot sit on a standard toilet wearing a catheter without having the tube constantly tugging against what you don't want it tugging against.

According to Wayne, who has never steered me wrong yet, sitting on one of the elevated seats—the ones with the armrests—alleviates that problem.

Lisa didn't find it necessary to follow Wayne's advice, but when I was able to sit on the toilet for the first time, I learned that Wayne Kinnett was a prophet. I pouted about that for a day and a half until our friend, Kathy Hope, showed up at the door with a brand new state-of-the-art hospital-style toilet seat. I wouldn't have appreciated her more if she had brought me a new Rolls-Royce.

I don't know how long day two lasted, but I know for a solid gold fact that it was a lot longer than twenty-four hours. But pass it did. When Lisa finally offered me that glorious combination of sleeping pill and pain pill at ten o'clock that night, I felt like the weight of the world was being lifted off my shoulders.

Honesty compels me to admit that when I woke up on the third day after surgery, the worst was behind me. I don't want to mislead you into thinking that it was all lightness and sunshine after that. I still had occasional bouts with excruciating pain caused by the build-up of gas in my stomach. I never did learn to get along well with my new companion, the Foley catheter. The first time I tried to take a shower with it, I stepped on the tube while stepping into the tub and almost pulled it out of own body, about a week ahead of schedule.

But I learned to cope. I began to take short walks outside. Every morning, for instance, I would walk up our long driveway to pick up the newspaper, carrying my urine bag in my hand. I must have looked like quite a sight to the motorists driving down Ebenezer Road. In the afternoons, I would walk around the farm, a few hundred yards at first. By the end of the week I was up to a half-mile.

My buddy, Gary, kept me company that week while Lisa went back to work. Gary was a Godsend. He is one of those rare friends who will accept you as you are—guts, feathers, and all. Gary spent a lot of hours sitting on the couch, watching television with the volume turned down, while I slept in my recliner on the other side of the room.

A few folks brought by food, although there was very little I could eat. Most of them just handed their trays to Lisa at the back door. Not many people seemed willing to walk into the lion's den and risk antagonizing the sleeping ogre that I must have been. Little by little, however, I began to feel human, although I knew I wouldn't really feel like a person again until the catheter was removed.

A funny thing happened about a day before that noteworthy event. At least it is funny now.

Eight months or so before my surgery, long before I would learn that I had cancer, I received a much-appreciated invitation to speak at the Sugar Hill Baptist Church Sportsmen Dinner. This is an annual event that serves as a sort of evangelistic outreach to men who might not show up for the typical church dinner or revival service. There were to be 600 folks in attendance and barbecue would be served. That engagement was right up my alley, understand, and I quickly accepted before the program committee had a chance to change its mind.

I wrote the date down on my calendar—August 25, 2011—and then didn't give it another thought. When, at the urging of Buddy Neel, I wrote about my impending surgery in the many newspapers that carry my column, I received a call from the good folks at Sugar Hill checking to make sure that I would be up to making a talk so soon after surgery. Dr. Miller had assured me that I would have the catheter out after ten days and would be up and around enough to "fake" feeling good after a couple of weeks. With the surgery on August 10 I was confident that I could speak on August 25.

Except I had written the wrong date on my calendar. I was scheduled to speak on August 18. Oops. There was no way I was going to cancel a gig that late no matter what the circumstances. I told the folks at Sugar Hill that I was looking forward to seeing them.

When that fateful Thursday arrived, I enlisted the help of my good friend, Bruce Walker. Bruce looks almost exactly like Kenny Rogers would look if he hadn't had work done. Bruce can also sing about as good as Kenny, too. I asked him to drive me up to Sugar Hill—about a one hundred mile round trip from Conyers—and prop me up long enough to say my piece. I figured if worse came to worse, I could just get Bruce to sing a little George Jones or Ferlin Huskey. The folks would enjoy that better anyway.

In order to make the trip, I had to take off my normal catheter bag—the one that I carried around on my arm like a purse—and wear the little strap-on, which fit under my pants, as long as I wore really baggy pants. The problem with the leg bag was that it didn't hold much urine and my body put out an awful lot of urine. We had to make frequent stops to empty my pants leg.

We arrived at the church without incident and I even managed to force down some really good barbecue. When it was almost time for me to go on, I popped a couple of Percocet tablets and made one last bathroom run. Bruce reminded me wryly that taking drugs in order to perform was what started Elvis on his downward spiral.

As I took the stage, I warned the audience that I was about a week removed from major surgery. I admitted that I had a catheter bag strapped to my leg under my pants, and then I said, "If I ask that every head be bowed and every eye closed, sho' 'nuff, y'all, I need every head bowed and every eye closed. I'll have a little adjusting to do."

I don't remember what I said after that, but it must have been pretty good stuff. As I tumbled into the car for the ride home, washing another Percoset down with a swallow of sweet tea, Bruce gave me the biggest compliment an old Sardis boy can give. He said, "You done good."

I must have, because I haven't known Bruce Walker to lie to me yet.

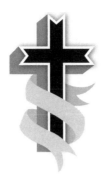

CHAPTER SEVENTEEN

It was about 8:30 p.m. on August 16. I remember that date because it was Elvis Day—the anniversary of the King of Rock and Roll's shocking death in Memphis.

I remember exactly where I was when I learned that Elvis had died. I was 25 and delivering furniture for Sam Ramsey as a part-time summer job—not to be confused with my full-time summer job, which was working at Bert Adams Boy Scout Reservation. My partner, Nolan Burrell, and I were making a delivery to Salem Campground. It was camp meeting week. After dropping off whatever it was we had dropped off at the Salem Hotel, we stopped at Gray's store, right across the road, to get a cold drink.

Everyone in the store was gathered around a small radio behind the counter. A couple of women were crying. "What happened?" I asked, wondering if there had been a political assassination or some other sort of man-caused tragedy.

"Elvis died," was the simple answer.

I was shocked and dismayed. Nolan, who was himself a musician and closer to Elvis' age, was distraught.

Nolan drove the furniture truck straight to the Ford place and had them install a radio. "They will be playing Elvis all weekend," he explained to me, as though having an unauthorized radio installed into the company truck made all the sense in the world. In a way, it did.

I always remember that story when August 16 rolls around and was, in fact, listening to an Elvis CD when the telephone rang in

August 2011. Dr. Miller was on the other end with great news. "Mark this down," he told me, "as the day you found out you are cancer-free!"

Now that was good news, indeed. He gave me the run-down on my pathology report. "Your prostate was in terrible shape" he told me. "The back side, especially, was almost mushy. But the capsule was intact, the margins were clean, the lymph nodes we tested were negative. It's all good. Your pathology report is clean as a whistle."

"Praise the Lord!" I exclaimed—or something like that. We talked for a while longer, me thanking him profusely for taking time to call with the good news. He confirmed the fact that I would be coming in a couple of days later for the blessed event of having my catheter removed. He casually mentioned that he would have his nurse draw some blood that day for a follow-up PSA test, just to be safe.

I thanked him again before we hung up and then I started calling everybody I knew to share the good news.

One of the people I called was Carole Denman. She used to be Carole Crawford and she was the friend who was with me when I was 18 and had the wreck that crushed my esophagus and started all the scar tissue and adhesion nonsense. Carole and I remained close friends throughout college and then sort of drifted apart like friends do.

She wound up married to a great guy named Steve Denman, who is a State Farm agent in Watkinsville, right outside Athens. A day or two after I wrote the column revealing I had prostate cancer, I got a call from Carole. She told me that Steve had prostate cancer, too, and that he would be seeing Dr. Miller about a week after my original consultation. Steve and I stayed about a week apart throughout the entire string of procedures that come with a prostatectomy. He was a great encouragement to me and it was nice to have someone to talk to throughout the whole ordeal that really understood.

I wanted to make sure he knew that my procedure worked so he could look forward to getting that same call soon. I am happy to report that he did.

I have had some mountaintop experiences in my life. I saw my children born. I've watched two of the three graduate from the University of Georgia, so far. Teams I have coached have won championships. I have enjoyed the thrill of having books published. On the first day of 1981, I watched the Georgia Bulldogs beat Notre Dame to become—in the words of the inimitable Dan Magill—the undefeated, untied, undisputed and undenied champions of college football. I have enjoyed some red letter days in my life.

None surpass the day Valerie removed my Foley catheter. It is a funny thing. As much as I looked forward to being without it, I really, really dreaded having it removed. I had almost removed it myself, you might recall, several times by stepping on it. At least that's what I thought. I never realized that there was a balloon inside me holding the catheter in place.

Valerie was as gentle as could be, and if you are ever facing a catheter removal, there is nothing to it. I mean it. She just pumped a lot of water into me so she could measure how much came out. Then she used a needle to deflate the balloon and told me to take a really deep breath and let it out, all at once. When I let my breath out, the catheter tube came too and the relief I felt more than made up for any slight pain I might have felt.

With the catheter gone and discarded, it was time to hear the stress continence talk. Men without prostate glands have to learn to hold their water all over again. Like women, they have to rely more on their muscles instead of their gland. For the first two or three months after a prostatectomy, virtually all men suffer from some degree of stress incontinence. That means they cannot control their urine output, especially during coughing, sneezing, breaking wind, or exercising. Sometime urine just pours out for the heck of it.

For some men this is a bigger problem than for others. A very small percentage, so I am told, experience permanent incontinence. Not me. Mine ended after three months, almost to the day Dr. Miller predicted it would. In the meantime, I had to deal with the dreaded incontinence pads. I now have great empathy for every woman I know, have known, or will ever know.

Valerie, after she removed my catheter, showed me how to use the pads and gave me enough to get home with. I thought the experience would be quite embarrassing, if not humiliating, but Valerie made sure that it was neither, bless her heart.

I was so relieved that the catheter was gone, even if I was wearing a maxi-pad and briefs instead of my normal boxers, I didn't even mind when she drew my blood, and I have been a baby about needles and blood-letting for as long as I can remember.

Lisa and I drove home happy that day, eager to get on with the rest of my life—and exceedingly thankful that there would be a rest of my life.

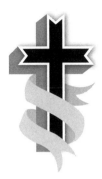

CHAPTER EIGHTEEN

I had never been so happy to welcome a month as I was September. I was sore and weak and tired—but I was alive and healing and eager to get well. I did everything I was told—or as close to it as I could and still be me. I enjoyed being at home and enjoyed, to a degree, being waited on. Every now and then I would have a visitor or two, and every day my inbox and snail-mail box was overflowing with cards and letters and well wishes. Everyone I knew went out of their way to let me know that they were sending up prayers on my behalf.

I appreciated each and every one of those prayers.

September brings college football, of course. I had mentioned to Dr. Miller that I really wanted to make it to the first Georgia game, against Boise State, in the Georgia Dome. It was September 3, three weeks and three days after my surgery. He didn't recommend it, but neither did he forbid it. I went. It was a disaster—for the Georgia team and for my health. Trent and Jeannine Goggins, two long-time friends, gave me a ride and we kept our walking to a minimum. It still took me three days to recover.

The next weekend was the big home opener against the Evil Genius, Steve Spurrier, and the South Carolina Gamecocks. I went over for the tailgate, but came home in time to watch the actual game on television. I am glad I did. I would not have survived the heated contest.

I finally made it inside the stadium when Deborah Dietzler, executive director of the UGA Alumni Society, invited me to enjoy the Mississippi State game from the air-conditioned confines of the Alumni Sky Box—far above the hallowed hedges of Sanford Stadium. Now that I know how the other half lives, I may be never be comfortable in Section 108 again.

Toward the end of September, I went back to school.

I first started teaching in 1974 at Cousins Middle School in Covington. I taught life science to seventh graders and coached middle school football and basketball. I stayed at Cousins for three years. It was the most satisfying three years of my career. I made relationships that are still strong today and it was at Cousins that I truly fell in love with teaching.

In 1999, after quite a winding path, I wound up teaching Advanced Placement U.S. History at Heritage High School—less than a mile from my home. I came to love teaching at Heritage. My wife had been in the first HHS graduating class in 1979. My in-laws had helped open the school and had both worked there for about a dozen years. All three of our children would graduate form Heritage. It had become home and, strange as it might sound, I couldn't wait to get back to school that September. I wanted to be around my many close friends there and I needed to be back around my students, who were amazing all year long. They gave me strength to go on when I didn't feel like going on.

I won't say that it was easy, though. I run what educational theorists call a teacher-centered class room. I use the Socratic method of instruction for the most part. It was good enough for Jesus. It is certainly good enough for me. I've never been one of those give-out-a-worksheet-and-sit-on-your-butt kinds of teachers. I've never been real big on group work, either. I firmly believe that I know more about history than any of my students and that I can teach them better than they can teach themselves. But it is hard to stand—or sit—for four or five hours a day and lead discussions or supervise students while they pursue assignments.

The first 90-minute period of the day wasn't bad. Second period was a little tougher. By the time the last class of the day arrived in my room, I was wasted. I was just "out of gas," as one of my students put it. But I persevered and my students persevered and we completed the year, one day at a time.

I had so much help from my fellow teachers and administrators and parents—words cannot describe how so many people helped sustain me. I was confident that I was well on my way to a full recovery.

Dr. Miller was great, by the way, throughout my whole recovery period about checking in from time to time to make sure I was doing OK and that my spirits were good. One evening, however, I got a somewhat disturbing call. He assured me that it was nothing to worry about, but the PSA test on the blood that Valerie had drawn wasn't exactly what he had wanted it to be. He was looking for a number somewhere below 1.0. Mine had come in at about 2.4.

"Everything will be fine," he assured me. If there were any concern in his voice, I could not detect it. He reminded me that my pathology report had been good. "We probably just drew the blood a little too soon," he said. "We'll wait a few weeks and then check it again."

Since he wasn't concerned, I tried not to be either. Things were going well. I was worn out at the end of each day, but I was walking a couple of miles each afternoon and had gone from eight to ten pads a day to five or six. I had only lost control of my bladder and soaked my pants once while at school. Luckily, I was behind my podium when that happened. If any students noticed, they pretended not to.

Besides, I had other fish to fry, if I might borrow a phrase from coaching genius Paul Johnson. I had to go back to Dr. Miller's office and see Curt. Or maybe it was Kirk. Anyway, I had to go and see the pump guy.

OK. We might be getting close to the realm of too much information, but it is a big part of the recovery process and far be it from me to allow modesty to prevent me from fully preparing a prospective cancer patient for what he might face. Besides, the whole thing is pretty funny, in an embarrassing sort of way.

"The Pump" refers to the Osbon ErecAid Esteem vacuum therapy system. One of the purposes of the device is to provide an immediate erection for men who cannot achieve one on their own. That was not why Dr. Miller prescribed the pump for me. When used regularly—meaning once a day—the pump is supposed to keep blood flowing into the right places on a regular basis so that once a man's nerve endings begin to function again after surgery, the blood vessels will be prepared to cooperate.

If I wanted anything, I wanted cooperative blood vessels, so I used the device faithfully, seven days a week, for months. I will spare you the details—you are welcome—but I made sure that the bathroom door was locked before I engaged in my therapy. Anyone who might have happened into the room would have been scarred for life. And there are people on our farm who—like my nephew, Tyler, when he was about four—have been known to wander into my bathroom.

I will leave this conversation with one observation. The pump hasn't worked out for me because of other complications, but my understanding is that it is of invaluable benefit to the sexual recovery for most post-op patients. So go see Curt. Or Kirk. Or whoever it is that sells the device these days.

Of course, the pump was supposed to be used in conjunction with medication, like Cialis or Levitra, which was to be taken not as needed, but every day or at least every other day. Therein lies the rub. There are at least 30 days in almost every month. (Speaking of which, can anybody really explain the whole February thing to me?) If you are going to take a pill every other day, you need at least 15 of those pills each month. Now understand, these pills were for therapy, to keep the old blood flowing. They were not being used for recreation. I wish they were, but they weren't. My insurance company allows the men it insures to "have fun" six times a month. I don't know who decided that six times a month is enough, but I bet it was a woman.

Honesty compels me to admit that if I were using the pills for fun, six a month would have been a gracious plenty. But I wasn't. And those things are expensive! We were spending a fortune on medication and I argued with the insurance people until I was blue in the face—among other places—but to no avail.

Having cancer is expensive, y'all. This is yet another reason to heed Wayne Kinnett's advice to avoid getting it.

At any rate, I survived September. Toward the middle of October, I went for the follow-up PSA test. Now we were sure that enough time had elapsed to ensure an accurate reading. Lisa fielded the phone call this time. The news was not good. The PSA had doubled.

"I think we are going to need a little radiation," was the doctor's verdict.

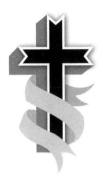

Chapter Nineteen

When I heard the news that, despite the fact that I no longer had a prostate gland, my PSA was climbing—and at an alarming rate—I thought back to a comment Scott Miller had made during our first encounter. Obviously sensing my discomfort and distress at having cancer, he looked at me with assurance and said, "You aren't going to die from this."

I took him at his word, for the most part, and throughout the surgery and recovery process, I considered my battle with cancer as an annoyance that had to be dealt with—a speed bump, albeit a rather high one—on the highway of life. Now, for the first time, I wasn't so sure. I went back to the place I had no business being—the internet.

What I found was disconcerting. Obviously, my cancer had escaped my prostate, probably long before my prostatectomy had been performed. I thought back to another comment Dr. Miller had made on August 16 when he called with the good news about the pathology report. "The prostate was mushy, as bad as I have ever seen. The Gleason score was higher on the pathology report than it had been on the autopsy. It was a Gleason 9."

None of that had mattered, of course, because it was preceded—and followed—by "the capsule was intact; the margins were clean."

What I learned on the internet—and what Dr. Miller would explain on my next visit—is that there is a particularly virulent strain of microscopic prostate disease that can escape into the blood without detection. The cells are so small that they are almost impossible to find. While the prognosis for most types of prostate cancer is good, especially with early detection, the odds decline dramatically if the cancer has unknowingly escaped into the blood prior to or just after surgery. The odds get worse if the cancer metastasizes—spreads to another organ or the bones. The odds get worse still if the PSA is doubling rapidly.

I didn't like anything I was reading.

The next step was a nuclear test called a Prostascint scan. This particular test took four days to complete. I had to travel up to North-side Hospital one day to be injected with radioactively tagged antibodies. These bad dudes have the unenviable task of traveling through the body, looking to attach themselves to prostate cancer cells. A few days later, I made the return trip and spent several hours under some sort of machine that could capture the images inside my body. They were looking for hot spots—places the antibodies had attached themselves—but didn't find any.

I suppose it was worth a shot, but we later found out that there is a certain degree of controversy over the value of the test. Some medical professionals belief it is a valid procedure. Others do not. My insurance company sided with those who do not and we are still trying to pay for that particular test. A word to the wise, here. Make sure everything is pre-certified.

Since we couldn't pinpoint the exact location of the cells that were loose inside my body, driving up my PSA, the radiation on-cologist Dr. Miller referred me to prescribed what I hoped would be my final treatment. He explained that the last known location of the prostate cancer was in the prostate, which was in the pelvis, before I had it removed. For forty days—not counting Saturdays, Sundays, and holidays—I would get five blasts of radiation throughout my pelvic area in hopes that the remaining cancer cells would be killed—graveyard dead—and I would be cured, once and for all.

My first visit to the radiation therapy clinic was on a cold and rainy day—the Monday before Thanksgiving—and the weather suited my mood perfectly. I couldn't help but laugh at the irony of the situation. When I was first diagnosed, my major concern was that

I would have to hang close to home for a month so that I could get radiation. Now I had been trying to recover from surgery for three months, and here I was waiting to begin not thirty days, but radiation treatments that would be spread out over two-and-a-half months because of the holidays.

A lot of people had tried to prepare me for what to expect during my treatments. I had been told that I would have my appointments at the same time every day and that everyone else would, too. I was assured that I would get to know my fellow patients really well and that we would form a close bond. Well, that didn't happen.

I was determined to teach every day. The way my class schedule worked, I could come for my treatments at 1:30 on some afternoons but not until 3:30 on others. Some days, however, I had out-of-town speaking engagements—particularly during the Christmas season—so I would come at 7 a.m. The folks that took care of me were very accommodating, but I seldom saw the same person more than once or twice. Most of the time they were exceedingly prompt, too—except for the first day.

I had all sorts of paperwork to fill out that day—with all sorts of embarrassing questions about my urinary habits, sexual performance—or lack thereof—and incontinence. I hated tell total strangers how many Depends pads I had to use each day. After I had turned in all my forms, I had to just sit there for what seemed like forever. Finally, one of the office folks came out and explained that their machine wasn't functioning properly. That's not what you want to hear—especially on your first day.

They had a technician working on it though. Now that was comforting. I could just see a guy resembling Goober Pyle from the Andy Griffith Show with his name embroidered above the pocket of his work shirt, banging on the radiation machine with a wrench and a hammer.

I was given the choice of waiting—but they didn't know for how long—or driving to Covington, ten miles away, and getting my first treatment there. With thoughts of Goober dancing in my brain, I opted for the Covington location. I drove through the rain, wondering what in the world I had gotten myself into, and finally found the clinic.

YEA THOUGH I WALK

It is funny, but I felt right at home there. A couple of people came up and introduced themselves. One was Amanda Hauptman, who happened to be the daughter of my lifelong friend, Dale Jeffries. Small world. My first thought upon meeting her was that it was one thing for a relatively old man like me to be battling cancer, but she was so young. I was reminded that cancer has no respect for age or gender or station in life; it is an equal opportunity killer.

Finally it was my turn to go back. I had been given a heads-up about the waiting room experience but had no idea what to expect once I got behind closed doors.

I was greeted in the back by three attractive young women who told me to pull down my pants and lie down on the treatment table. I must have looked embarrassed because one of them handed me a cocktail napkin and said, "You can cover up with this."

I looked at the diminutive scrap of paper and said, "Don't you have anything bigger?" I was hoping for at least a dinner napkin.

"That's big enough," she assured me. Sadly, she was right.

Next, they swung this huge machine over me that looked like a death ray from the old Buck Rogers comic books. Then they started shining lasers all over my pelvic region and a young woman came in and started drawing all kinds of crazy shapes—ovals, rectangles, squares, circles—all over my body with an indelible Sharpie. I looked like one of those crash dummies you used to see on the television commercials. When she had gotten me all marked up she swapped her Sharpie for a needle and started tattooing my body. I asked for a mermaid, but didn't get one.

Once I had been properly prepped, the ladies all went behind a lead shield and turned on the radiation. I got about a thirty second dose—just guessing here because they made me take off my watch—and then the machine rotated to another spot before giving me the next dose. I got zapped five times in all. Then they told me to get dressed and sent me on my way.

The next day, I went back to the Conyers location and had to disrobe in front of three more total strangers. This visit was shorter, however, because I already had my tats and other markings. I would come back the next day and then take five days off to celebrate Thanksgiving. We would begin again on the following Monday.

This pattern would continue into the middle of February. I got to know my primary technicians, Vi and Bernadette, extremely well and they were wonderful—caring and professional and personable—I actually came to look forward to the ten or fifteen minutes I spent with them every day, lying on their table and getting lit up like a Christmas tree notwithstanding.

Just before I was about to have my first treatment, Bob Bradley, a lifelong friend and current assistant principal at my school, told me that he had read a story about baseball great Tony Gwynn, who had undergone radiation for a different type of cancer. Gwynn, in the article, commented on a bell that was on the counter of his treatment facility. Upon completion of the treatment cycle, patients were urged to ring the bell loud and long to celebrate that they had surpassed a milestone in their personal war with cancer. Gwynn said that thinking about ringing that bell kept him coming back for treatments day after day.

They had a bell at my facility, too. After about my second time on the table with Vi and Bernadette, I started counting down the days until I could pick that sucker up and make it peal. As that great day approached, I wrote a column about the bell. Folks tell me that on the day of my last treatment bells were ringing from Rabun Gap to Tybee Light—including the venerable old Chapel Bell on the UGA campus. My buddy Dennis Fifield even brought me a genuine cowbell, which I now keep on my desk at school to remind me of that stage of my journey.

If, heaven forbid, you or yours are ever faced with undergoing radiation therapy, don't let anyone tell you that it is easy. It is not. It zaps your energy—I stayed worn out the entire time I was taking the radiation—and it has side effects. Let's just say that I really did feel like celebrating when I knew I didn't have to climb on that table again.

A couple of weeks after my last treatment, I went in for yet another PSA test. After having my blood drawn, I met with the doctor at the clinic to learn what the results of the test would tell us. She told me that they were hoping that the PSA level would be less than .2. That's not less than 2, a whole number integer, understand—but .2—a very minute fraction. That would let us know that the therapy had worked and that the cancer had, finally, been nipped in the bud—to quote the immortal Barney Fife.

Then she added, and I will never forget this comment—"If, heaven forbid, the number is something like 1.8, well, then"—and her voice trailed off before she added—"I don't know what we would do then."

I thanked her and went home to begin the long four-day wait to hear my results. They call finally came from the lab. My PSA was not less than .2. And it was higher than 1.8. It was closer to a 7, which is not a really high number, except that my PSA had practically doubled during my forty days of radiation.

Now it was time to worry.

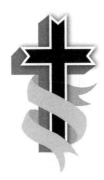

CHAPTER TWENTY

I know I didn't deal with my cancer as well as some people do, but I did the best I could. When all is said and done, that is all any of us can really do. The great philosopher, Herschel Walker, once said—at the tender age of eighteen—"Well, I don't know what people expect out of me, but what they are going to get is all I got; I hope they don't expect more than that because if they do, they will be disappointed."

What people got out of me from November until February was all I had. Sometimes that was pretty good. Sometimes it wasn't very good at all.

When most people asked me how I was doing—and lots and lots of people asked me how I was doing—I simply smiled and said, "Fine, how're you?" When people asked me how I was doing—and I really thought they wanted to know—I would tell them. Those folks heard a lot of whining and a lot of despair on the bad days and a lot of hope on the good days.

During the Thanksgiving season, when I was still confident that the radiation would do its job, I was upbeat and spent a lot of time counting a long list of blessings, and make no mistake, I have been genuinely blessed by God Almighty. When an old boy from Porterdale gets to do the things I've done and go the places I've been and have the family that I have, he has been blessed exceedingly. "My cup runneth over."

YEA THOUGH I WALK

During Christmas, though, I became a bit morose. The radiation was wearing me down and when I got caught up in the emotions of the season, I would wonder if this would be my last Christmas. Christmas always makes me a little melancholy, anyway. I think about the many happy holiday seasons I have spent with those who have passed on and who are no longer here with me and it makes me sad—sad that they aren't still here and sad that I didn't appreciate them enough when they were.

I also get frustrated at Christmas because I can never seem to find the right gifts for my kids and Lisa, gifts that are meaningful and show them just how much I really love them. On the first Christmas, God gave the world his only begotten son to die for all our sins. God set the bar pretty high on that first Christmas, as far as gift-giving goes.

Now understand, my kids don't expect expensive and elaborate material things. They realize that relationships and time together are the most important part of the yuletide celebration. I'm the one who wants to find them spectacular gifts—and I always feel that I fall short.

My mama, now, she could come up with a great gift in a pinch. I remember the Christmas after my daddy died. She knew that I really missed him and that Christmas was a lonely time for me that year. She wanted to give me a really special present. She did, too. She made me the most beautiful red, white and blue starburst quilt that anyone has ever seen. I knew that she had put unconditional love into every stitch and I will treasure that quilt until the day I die. I just hope that whoever winds up with the quilt after that will treasure it as much as I do.

We did get through Christmas without any major breakdowns. I gave my kids television sets and autographed Pat Conroy books. Not exactly handmade quilts. Doesn't approach a savior for the world, but like I said earlier—I did my best.

Mostly during this period of time, I just tried to keep on keeping on. I continued getting up early on Wednesday mornings and trying to make people laugh at my "What the Huck" spot on the Moby in the Morning Show. I made dozens of speeches and personal appearances during this time—at churches, conventions, conferences and goat roping. "Have mouth, will travel," was my motto. I was just like Paladin except with a Dodge Caravan instead of a horse. I wrote four columns a week. And I continued to teach school.

I got a lot of inspiration at school from a lot of people.

Caroline Ingle was at school, for instance. Caroline is the daughter of Wayne and Carol Ingle of Conyers. They were Miss and Mr. Rockdale County High School together, back in the previous century, and childhood sweethearts. Wayne played football on Vince Dooley's first three teams at the University of Georgia and was on the field during the 1965 Alabama game—so he says—when Pat Hodgson replaced him, bringing in the historic flea-flicker play that allowed Georgia to beat Alabama and the legendary Bear Bryant 18-17 in 1965.

I love Bear Bryant. He's the only football coach in America to ever have an animal named after him.

I love Caroline, too. We go way back. I taught her Sunday school class when she was in the eighth grade and I learned a lot from her. When she taught in a mission school in South Central Los Angeles, Lisa and I went out to visit her. I spent two days in her classroom and realized then what a gifted teacher she was. Later, she would come to work at Heritage High School in Conyers, and she has let her light shine here just as brightly as she had on the left coast.

On Labor Day weekend in 2010, Caroline was diagnosed with leukemia. She was 34. For a solid year, our entire community wore orange—the color for leukemia cancer support. Caroline and her whole family fought with every ounce of strength in their bodies—and won. Now Caroline is cancer free. Time after time during that awful winter I would turn to Caroline for strength and advice and encouragement and she never once let me down. "Always there for me" is an overused term—but Caroline was always there for me.

Linda Moore was an inspiration, too. Linda taught English right down the hall from me. I always said that when I got to school and saw Linda in the halls that I knew the Rapture had not occurred. I might have been left behind, but Linda Moore wouldn't be. Linda was 65 and fighting a plethora of health problems of her own. She had to go to kidney dialysis several time a week. Eventually, she would have to navigate the halls of our school in a wheelchair. I know that she was fatigued and in great pain, but she was there every day. She asked no quarter of her disease. Many, many days when I didn't feel like being at school I knew that Linda felt worse. I just got up and came on.

Linda would suffer a stroke in February and go to be with the Lord in June, but she still inspires me and I think about her every day.

The school administration and my fellow teachers were wonderful. My principal, Greg Fowler, an old Prattville, Alabama, boy, never even blinked when I needed to be gone for a doctor's appointment or a treatment. If I needed to go the house and rest during my planning period—I live within a mile of the school—I went to the house and rested, no questions asked. Of course, he might wake me up with a text at ten o'clock at night wanting to know something about the 1966 Georgia gubernatorial race or how old Uga III was when he died, but he left me alone at school.

Miss Lizzie, the lady who had cleaned my room for me every day for fifteen years, had a hug for me every morning and a prayer for me every afternoon. Some days she would send me home as soon as my classes were over. I love Miss Lizzie for caring so much.

Naturally, I will get in trouble if I start naming names, because I can't name them all, but, really—everyone was great. Dave LaBarrie, the assistant principal in charge of social studies at our school; Bob Bradley, whose father was my high school coach,; boy wonder Marion Hanahan, our social studies department chair; Peggy Hanahan, his mother—who really ran things—they all bent over backwards to make my life as easy as life can be when you teach eleventh graders for a living.

Poor Harry Duke. I knew that when I was feeling really bad and needed somebody to unload on, I could unload on Harry. I could tell him exactly how I was feeling and be as gruff as I wanted to be and he never took it personally.

Scott Wade, one of my favorite people in the world, would come into my classroom during his planning period several days a week.

He claimed he was there to observe and learn and to be entertained, but I know he was there so he could take over if I got past going.

Scott Foster was another trooper. He is in charge of technology at our school and is a huge Georgia fan. One thing has little to do with the other, but I couldn't mention Scott without a shout out to the Dawgs. When his phone rings, it plays Glory, Glory and he stops whatever he is doing to salute. I know very little about technology. I have a 21st Century Classroom with thousands of dollars worth of bells and whistles and computers and media but I have a 20th century mind. I didn't have to worry. If I needed anything at all, Scott got it done before I knew I needed him to do it. He was like Radar O'Reilly on M.A.S.H.

I have to back up and say another word about the Hanahans. They are from Dothan, Alabama, and are such huge Crimson Tide fans that they believe that if you are good, when you die you go to Nick Saban's house. Marion can't wait.

I know. I'm a thief. Lewis Grizzard said that about Dorsey Hill. Speaking of which, Dorsey Hill even called me a couple of times while I was real sick. If I had heard from Lewis, I would have really worried.

Peggy Hanahan taught at Dothan High School for a quarter of a century and then retired from the Alabama public school system and came to work at Heritage about a dozen years ago. Their loss was our gain. I would talk to Peggy when I didn't want to talk to anyone. I knew I could be frank with her and tell her when I was tired or in pain or afraid. She never judged. She always listened. She always understood. Everybody who has cancer needs a Peggy Hanahan in his or her life.

Five years ago Peggy's son, Marion, joined us at Heritage and is a rising star in the field of public education. He has already been named Teacher of the Year for our county and will soon be Dr. Marion Hanahan. Two years ago, he became our department chair, mostly by default, but still. He worried more about me than my own kids did and gave me daily encouragement and treated me like my well-being was the most important item on his daily agenda. I will never forget him for that.

He will never forget me—or perhaps the word is forgive me, either.

Marion is a huge Alabama fan. Huge. He loves Alabama so much that he risked his job a couple of years ago by missing the start of the second semester to fly to Pasadena to watch the Tide play Texas in the Rose Bowl for the BCS Championship. I wouldn't say that I encouraged such unprofessional behavior, but I did buy his plane ticket for him while he was still at the Georgia Dome watching his team win the SEC championship game.

Actually, he was never in danger of losing his job either. Greg Fowler, our principal, is an Alabama alum, too. He understands.

But I was explaining why Marion might never forgive me for messing up his life. He had a girlfriend—a really pretty girlfriend, too. There was just one problem. She was a Yankee—from Chicago. It may have been Indiana but Chicago makes a better story. Actually, New Jersey would make an even better story, but I know she wasn't from Jersey.

I was concerned for my boy's future happiness. I know how he is during football season—and spring football season. I knew this young lady, as pretty as she was, would never understand his passion for the game and those mixed marriages just never work out. I told him that he should ask the girl if she knew how many points a safety counts in football. If she said "two" then I gave him the green light to proceed with the romance, but if she didn't know, I suggested he give her the rest of the year off.

He took my advice and asked her. She didn't have a clue. They were done.

I sincerely hope I haven't impeded his future happiness.

Mike Beshiri was an encourager, too, because most people think that Mike, a gruff old retired army colonel who teaches German as a second career, was either born without a heart or lost his at an early age. Those of us who know him best realize that nothing could be further from the truth.

I know Mike about as well as anyone. We were Scout leaders together and spent a week as bunkmates in a 5-foot-by-7-foot tent at Camp Rainy Mountain one summer when our kids were Tenderfoot Scouts in Troop 83. You learn a lot about a guy when you tent together. I learned not to serve him boiled chicken for supper, I can tell you that.

We also coached soccer together for several years. The other coaches hated us because we won almost every game. This was youth soccer, understand, and every kid had to play a certain number of minutes. We went out of our way to make sure everybody got plenty of playing time. We did. But Mike is a very competitive person, so a couple of times, against really good teams, he accidentally told the least skilled player on our team that game started about an hour-and-a-half after it really did. That particular kid would come running down to the sideline just as time expired. Bless his heart.

I am not about to reveal his name. I don't think he ever caught on and I'm not about to rat out Beshiri because the kid is now a sheriff's deputy in our community.

I knew I shouldn't have started this. There were so many prayer warriors, like Jason Price, who would make the long walk down from the ninth grade hall of our school on a daily basis just to let me know he was lifting my name on high, and Drew Williams. Drew and I have a lot of mutual acquaintances. I am one of many who helped him find his bride, Kelli, and he has helped me make a lot of connections around Northeast Georgia. Drew and I can't talk about politics or college football, but we talked a lot about the prayers he was saying on my behalf.

I can't leave this subject without telling you about Jim Hauck.

Jim teaches the history of the whole world to the same tenth graders that I get in the eleventh grade. I like Jim a lot. I really do. I don't like him quite as much as I like his wife, Judy, but I like Jim. He's a Georgia man. and although he was born in New York, he has adapted well to the American South. There's just one thing about Jim. He is slightly to the left of Nancy Pelosi, politically.

Don't ask me why. I have no explanation.

There's a big joke around town that Jim spent a whole year trying to make the students believe in his liberal causes and then I spend the first week of the next year getting their thinking straightened out. The funny thing is, the kids think we are sworn enemies—mostly,

I suppose, because he makes cracks about my political views all year and I return the favor the next year.

I will never forget the time my daughter Jenna's friend, Nadia, was having supper with us and I mentioned something Jim, Judy, Lisa and I had done when we were vacationing together in California. She almost swallowed a biscuit whole. "You and Coach Hauck go on vacation together? I thought you hated one another!"

We still laugh about that.

Tony Gray—the Sage of Salem Road—you will hear about later, and to the fellow teachers and friends I have failed to mention by name, I love you all, too.

In early January, when I was halfway through the radiation treatment and really struggling, Jim was waiting for me in front of my classroom door and asked me if I would walk down to his room and take a look at a project he was working on. We trudged around to his side of the building. He unlocked the door and I walked into his room. It was full of kids wearing red and black T-shirts with a "We Love Huck" logo on the front. On the back was my favorite classroom expression, "Hark a Lark!"

I felt a thousand feet high and those kids wore those shirts the rest of the year. I don't think a day went by that I didn't see at least one of the shirts strolling down the hall or sitting in my classroom.

I later learned that Jim, in cahoots with Julie Kimble, our English department chair and another great supporter, and some of my students, had secretly ordered the shirts. Of course they wanted them to say "Huck Off Cancer," but Greg Fowler, wanting to remain principal at Heritage, vetoed that one.

There are many other people I could tell you about at Heritage High School, including every one of my students, but you get the picture. A lot of people couldn't believe that I kept teaching through the year. There wasn't a better place for me to spend my days.

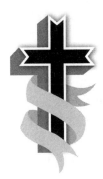

CHAPTER TWENTY-ONE

They say that confession is good for the soul. Methinks my soul is about to feel a whole lot better because I have a few to make. It won't be easy.

I used to have a good friend named Mo Akin. Mo and I went to church together at Ebenezer United Methodist Church. Mo and his wife, Mary, who was one of the best cooks ever born in the American South—and that means the world—have gone on to be with the Lord now. I still miss them. The people at Ebenezer still miss them, too, and once a year I know they miss Mo's barbecue and Brunswick stew, because he was a master at those and served as the chief cook at the Ebenezer barbecue for as long as I knew anything about it.

Mo always was one to speak his mind on matters of the church. I like that in a person. He was also one to give a compliment whenever he could. He lived in our general neighborhood and drove by my house just about every day of his life after we moved to Conyers. During the summer months, he used to tell me every Sunday, "I drove by your house this week. Your yard sure does look good from the road."

If Mo ever drove down our long driveway and got a close-up look at our yard, he might have been in for a surprise and he might have been singing a different tune on Sunday morning. Yes, our yard usually did look good from the road. The lawn was green and the shrubs were full and the flowers were colorful—we always put out a lot of flowers in our yard.

But we are about 150 yards off the road. Upon closer inspection, though, a person might get a different picture. To this day we haven't been able to cultivate a lawn free of weeds. Have you ever seen one of those before and after commercials for weed killer? The before picture has dandelions and crab grass and every broadleaf weed known to man. They used our yard for that picture.

When I kept the grass cut low, the weeds looked the same as the Bermuda grass from the road. But that was from the road. Our flowerbeds usually needed weeding, too, and the walk always needed trimming. The shrubs were often eaten up with aphids and don't even get me started on the gopher holes and pine straw beds. Yes, our yard looked good from the road but not nearly as good close up.

You might have noticed that I used the past tense to describe our yard. Truth be known, I should have used the present tense because our yard still looks pretty much the same—up close. The thing is though, that for a long, long time, my walk with God was a lot like our yard. It looked good from a distance, but upon closer examination, it left a lot to be desired.

There hasn't been a day in my life since I learned to create conscious thought that I didn't love Jesus or know that He loved me. I was raised in the church—my mama used to say that I was a Methodist for nine months before I was born—and accepted Christ as my savior at a very early age. It wasn't put on. I have always known and loved Jesus. I haven't always lived in His will, however. I have often been just too stubborn to give myself over to God completely. I have always tried to stay in control of my own life.

The Bible says that a man must not have two masters because he will love the one and hate the other. I wanted to be the master of my own fate. I tried to serve God while marching to the beat of my own drum. From the road, it looked like it was working; but in reality, not so much. I was often angry and bitter and could never be satisfied with the ways things went at church or the way things went at home or the way things went in my personal life.

Don't hear something I am not saying. I wasn't living a double life or putting on a charade. I prayed to God and was sincere. I went to church and my worship was genuine. I traveled around the country and spoke of the goodness of God and meant every word I ever uttered. I was as nice as I could be and I tried to help folks that needed helping and did my best to live out God's commandments. But that wasn't all God wanted from me and I knew that wasn't all. Because I wasn't willing—or able—to give myself completely to Him, I was always just a little bit out of sync with myself. There were times when I felt like one of those lukewarm Christians that Jesus wants to spit out of his mouth.

When I was diagnosed with cancer, I began immediately to add healing for myself to my daily prayer list and was confident that God would hear my prayers and heal me. I never doubted it for a second. Honesty compels me to admit, however, that when I learned that the operation hadn't worked and the radiation hadn't worked, I was absolutely despondent when left in the privacy of my own thoughts. I began to think about all the years I had wasted by not following more closely in Christ's footsteps, by not striving more earnestly for perfection in my everyday life. I would lie down at night to say my prayers and my body would ache—I wasn't just tired; I was weary. There is a difference. Lots of nights I would try to pray and the words would just not come. I was so heart sick and so soul sick that I couldn't form the words I needed to say in my own mind, much less make them come out of my mouth.

On those long nights I would rely on simple prayers and Bible verses that I had learned as a child. Many, many nights, when I was so weary and in so much pain that I didn't believe there was any way I could live through the night, all I could find strength to do was utter the prayer my parents had led me in before I went to sleep in our little four-room mill house those many, many years before.

"Now I lay me down to sleep, I pray the Lord my soul to keep. If I should die before I wake, I pray the Lord my soul to take." And then, yes, I would. I would start on a long litany of folks who were important to me that I hoped God would truly bless.

"God bless Mama and Daddy," and images of my parents would flood my brain, and without being able to form the words, even in my mind, I would hope that God knew I was giving him thanks for allowing me to have two such wonderful parents who loved me and sacrificed for me and taught me right from wrong.

"God bless Myron and Steve—and David and Rodney." My sister and her husband have been so good to me and so supportive of my endeavors, and so proud of me. I have done a poor job of showing them how much I love them and respect them. They have had a lot of tough breaks over the years and I have never done an adequate job of giving them comfort during hard times. I told you I was going to confess some things.

Myron wanted to help so much during the worst periods of my illness, but I didn't know how to let her. She wanted to hear about what I was going through every day and offer her support, but I didn't want to talk about it, to her or anyone else. I hoped that by asking blessings on her and Steve, God would somehow interpret how I felt about them.

"God bless Jamie, Jackson, and Jenna." I wasn't sure how my cancer was affecting my children. We've never been a family that talks about feelings—not in depth. I knew—and know—that they love me, just as I love them, but I didn't know how to tell them that my greatest fear while dealing with this disease was that I would die before finding out that they were well on the way to happy, prosperous, and Godly lives.

Every night for years—ever since he had told me that he was changing his major to education—I had prayed that Jackson would find a good job in a school in which he could actually teach children that want to learn, a school in which he would be appreciated for all of his good qualities. Such a situation is very rare in today's educational climate and growing rarer with each passing semester. Jackson Lee Huckaby—who was named after that Jackson and that Lee—is the best man I know. He embodies the positive character traits of the two great Southerners for whom he was named and I want him to have the purpose-filled life he deserves.

I prayed that my daughter Jamie Leigh, who is smart, beautiful, and loves life—and the Georgia Bulldogs—would find the person that God has had in mind for her since the creation of the earth to share her life. And I prayed that Jenna would survive being Jenna, that she would also find her intended mate, that she would take time to rest, that she would somehow tame her inner Towanda and physically survive her thrill-seeking lifestyle, and that God would continue to use her to glorify His name.

That's a lot for God to get out of "God bless Jamie, Jackson, and Jenna"—but He did. As this book goes to press, Jackson has secured the best teaching position in the history of education, at North Oconee High School in Watkinsville. No, he didn't have to leave Athens and I am not sure he ever will.

We are busy planning Jamie's wedding, and her fiancé, Chris, is a good ol' boy, a Georgia graduate and soon to be a practicing attorney—but I like him anyway.

And Jenna—well, so far she has survived being Jenna and continues to provide the light of Christ to a dark world.

God bless Benny and Bitzi. They are Lisa's parents and the only parents I've known for fourteen years. Everyone knows that I married way up and Benny and Bitzi are two of the reasons why.

God bless Mama and Daddy. My own parents have been gone a long time, but I still give thanks every day for the way they raised me and the unconditional love they always showed me.

God bless Eddie and Terry Lynn and Tyler and Maegan—Lisa's brother and his family who live right across the pasture. We don't spend as much time with them as we should, but we sure know where to find them if we need them—and they, I hope, know where to find us.

I would go on and on and on, until I drifted off to sleep, wondering if I would see morning. So far I haven't missed a one.

Eventually, as I gained more control of my emotions, I was able to follow up my simple childish prayers by reciting Bible verses I had memorized as a small child. The one that came most readily, and seemed to best fit my circumstances, was the prayer of the shepherd boy who killed a giant. Every night and many, many times a day, I would recite to myself—and often aloud—Psalms 23.

YEA THOUGH I WALK

The Lord is my shepherd; I shall not want.
He maketh me to lie down in green pastures:
he leadeth me beside the still waters.
He restoreth my soul: he leadeth me in the paths of
righteousness for his name's sake.
Yea, though I walk through the valley of the shadow of death,
I will fear no evil: for thou art with me;
thy rod and thy staff they comfort me.
Thou preparest a table before me in the presence of mine
enemies: thou anointest my head with oil; my cup runneth over.
Surely goodness and mercy shall follow me all the days of my life:
and I will dwell in the house of the Lord forever.

I learned the 23rd Psalm from the King James Bible, and as I lay in bed each night, filled with such anguish that my mind would not formulate new words and sentences of my own, I recited it as a prayer to God in the King James vernacular. I am still doing so several times a day.

Sometimes I would recite the Apostle's Creed, too, just to remind myself what I really believe in—and to make sure God realized that I still believe.

"I believe in God, the Father Almighty, maker of heaven and earth, and in Jesus Christ, his only begotten son, our Lord. Conceived by the Holy Spirit, born of the Virgin Mary, suffered under Pontius Pilate. He was crucified, dead and buried. The third day he arose from the dead. He ascended into heaven and sitteth at the right hand of God, the Father Almighty. From thence He shall come to judge the quick and the dead. I believe in the Holy Spirit, the holy catholic church, the communion of saints, the forgiveness of sins, the resurrection of the body and the life, everlasting."

I always followed that with the Lord's Prayer.

Eventually I was able to make it through this litany every night, and as I reminded myself of these universal truths that have been the foundation of my faith life since I have been old enough to walk and talk, I began to find a degree of peace that I hadn't had in a long time. I would repeat the litany every morning and search the Bible for words of encouragement and promises of hope. The book is full of both, you know.

And talk about God-instances! Every day—every single day—I would find passages that seemed to have been written just for me and my situation. That's because they were, of course. Let me give you a for-instance.

On one of the worst days I had, a morning after a long night of pain and weeping and agony and sleeplessness, I turned randomly to the Psalms 6. Let me share it with you, from the NIV:

Lord, do not rebuke me in your anger
or discipline me in your wrath.
Have mercy on me, Lord, for I am faint;
heal me, Lord, for my bones are in agony.
My soul is in deep anguish.
How long, Lord, how long?
Turn, Lord, and deliver me;
save me because of your unfailing love.
Among the dead no one proclaims your name.
Who praises you from the grave?
I am worn out from my groaning.
All night long I flood my bed with weeping
and drench my couch with tears.
My eyes grow weak with sorrow;
they fail because of all my foes.
Away from me, all you who do evil,
for the Lord has heard my weeping.
The Lord has heard my cry for mercy;
the Lord accepts my prayer.
All my enemies will be overwhelmed with shame and anguish;
they will turn back and suddenly be put to shame.

Don't waste your time trying to tell me that wasn't written for me, 3,500 years ago.

Gradually my spiritual life became stronger and stronger again as I was reminded of God's goodness and righteousness. I began to explore the Bible more deeply every day, reminding myself of Biblical truths that have been the foundation of my life for decades.

I continued with my personal liturgy every night—minus the "Now I lay me down to sleep" part—but now I followed the ritual with long conversations with God. I spent a lot of time praising him for his creation and thanking him for the innumerable gifts with which he has blessed me. The more I proclaimed, the more I remembered. I confessed—and repented—of my many, many sins, and I continued to pray for so many other people—all the folks I know who are hurting and suffering and fighting battles of their own. The more I prayed for others, the less I worried about myself. I continued to ask God for healing, and with each passing day, I gained confidence that I would truly be healed. I proclaimed to God that as I was being healed, I would use my illness in whatever way I could to bring glory and honor to His holy name. And I promised that, once healed, I would do everything in my power to live continuously in His will and do everything I could to become the man He created me to be.

My body continued to ail, but day by day, but I was getting right with God, which is a lot more important than weeding the flower bed or killing crabgrass.

My yard still looks pretty bad up close, but up close or at a distance, by and by, things would become more than well with my soul. I would find that perfect peace that passes all understanding. It would be a long walk, however.

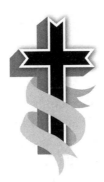

CHAPTER TWENTY TWO

Once we got over the shock of learning that the radiation had not worked and that my cancer had obviously escaped the prostate gland, probably before I even had surgery, we started looking around for the next option. Plan A had not worked. Plan B had not worked. We were prepared to go through the entire alphabet to Plans X, Y, Z, and start over at A if we had to—and by "we" I mean myself, my lovely wife, Lisa, and all of the prayer warriors we had enlisted along the way.

Let me say a word about those prayer warriors. I know for a fact that they were legion. I personally heard from thousands of people—and though I am prone to exaggeration, I am not exaggerating this time—who said they prayed for me every day. I received more than a hundred church bulletins with my name on the weekly prayer list. Every prayer was appreciated and every prayer was heard by God—of this I am certain. Every prayer helped and every time I heard that another person was praying for me, I was encouraged and my spirits were lifted.

I was asked by so many people, "What can I do?"

My answer was always, "Please pray for me," and I asked that unashamedly. I am not one to ask people to do things for me and I have a hard time accepting gifts and favors, but I was eager to have prayers.

We weren't going to rely solely on prayer, however. I believe that God has given us doctors and medical research for a reason and we intended to take advantage of every medical professional at our disposal.

The day we went to our oncologist to discuss the options after learning of the elevated PSA score following radiation, we stopped by Conyers Pharmacy to refill a prescription. Our daughter, Dr. Jamie, came out from behind the counter where she fills prescriptions each day to hear what the doctors had told us. As Lisa was telling her the news and going over the steps we intended to take, Jamie mumbled three words, almost under her breath. When Lisa paused to take a breath, I asked Jamie what she had said.

"M.D. Anderson," she repeated.

"Do what?" I responded.

"You should go to M.D. Anderson," she replied. "It is the best cancer center in the world and they are the most aggressive at treating all types of cancers. You need to go there."

Lisa interjected that we didn't really need to go there. She insisted that there were doctors at Emory who were just as good and pointed out that Clifton Road was a lot closer and a lot more accessible than Houston, Texas.

I had never really heard of M.D. Anderson, but I tended to agree with Lisa. I had always heard great things about Emory and personally know lots and lots of people they had helped tremendously. They had recently helped save the life of my friend Caroline, for instance. I wanted to give them a try, and we did.

Let me say this right now. I still believe in Emory and I still believe that we are really fortunate to have such a fine institution in our area. Thank God and Coca-Cola for Emory University Hospital. I just didn't feel after our visit that Emory was the place for me to pursue my treatment.

We called Emory and were able to get an appointment with the doctor we wanted to see. That was a positive. Our appointment was for 4:30 in the afternoon.

We sort of knew our way around Emory, so we found a parking place and made our way to the correct location without too much trouble. That's a bigger thing than it may sound like because Lewis and Clark we ain't.

I have sat in enough doctors' waiting rooms over the past year and a half to last me the rest of my life. Well, I suppose that's not such a good statement. Suffice it to say that I have seen my share and most of them are very depressing for various reasons. This one was no different, only more so.

We were finally called back to an examination room and I sat there nervously, anxious to hear words of hope from the doctor we were about to see. There was a rap on the door and I looked up expectantly as the nurse walked in, tossing a chart onto the table next to the door. She smiled at me and said, "OK, you are free to go."

"Go where?" I asked her, completely befuddled.

"Home," she answered, "or anywhere you want to go. You are all done."

"All done?" I countered. "We just got here. We haven't even seen anyone, yet."

I got a very quizzical look from the nurse who picked up the chart and examined it. Then, looking back at me, "You are Mr. Wilson aren't you?"

"No," I shook my head, "I am Mr. Huckaby."

"Oh," was the only response I got as she sashayed out the door.

A few minutes later, a different nurse came in, holding—I hoped—a different chart.

"Mr. Huckaby?" she inquired.

Now we were getting somewhere. "That's me," I answered.

She barely glanced at me, but rather gave her attention to Lisa. "Your dad really looks good for his age," she told her, as if I weren't even in the room.

Lisa gets that "dad" thing a lot, I am sorry to say—but not as sorry as she probably is. She just shrugs it off, as she did this time.

Not me, though. "I'm her husband," I corrected her. This statement elicited a really surprised look.

"OK," she said. Not, "Oh, of course. I'm sorry." Just "OK."

Then she started asking me questions. "You were born on March 10?"

"Yes," I replied.

"1915?" she asked.

139

"1915?" I parroted.

"Yes," she responded. "Is your birthday March 10, 1915?"

"Lord," I thought, "Do I really look 97?" I didn't ask her that, however, because I was afraid she'd say yes.

"No," I told her. "I was born in 1952. I am 60, not 100."

She didn't even look embarrassed. She simply said, "Oh, I guess I should have realized that was wrong."

My confidence wasn't exactly growing at this point.

She asked me a few more questions, scribbled something on my chart and then left us with the promise that "the doctor will be in shortly."

He was.

Now let me say this. First and foremost, I choose doctors for their knowledge and expertise. I had researched this particular doctor. He had all the right degrees from all the right schools and his credentials were impeccable. I also want a doctor that I can communicate with, one that will understand me and my background. I think that is important because I want a doctor who can understand and relate to my fears and anxieties. Other folks might not believe this to be important whatsoever. I am not trying to describe the experiences and thought processes of other folks. I am describing mine.

I did not click with this particular doctor. He did not ask me any personal questions or take a nanosecond of his valuable time to ask me about my thoughts or feelings. He had me lean over the table while he donned a rubber glove and gave me a manual examination to make sure my surgeon hadn't "left any of the prostate behind"—pun not intended.

I had hoped that the one positive of having my prostate removed would be that I would never have to have such an examination again, and told him so—adding that Scott Miller was my surgeon and I am certain he didn't leave any of my prostate gland behind.

"I don't know Scott Miller," he replied, quite caustically, "so I am going to check for myself."

I was offended. How did he not know Scott Miller? I knew for a fact that my doctor was the guru of robotic prostate surgery. How did this guy not know him? For the next fifteen or twenty minutes, our guy told us that the things we had done to date were not the right things to have done. He also spent a lot of time telling us how he was going to knock my PSA down and that he was going to do this and he was going to do that—with very little reference to my role in this little drama. I got the impression that my prostate cancer was merely an opportunity for him to exhibit his knowledge and skills. If I sound critical, I guess I am. As I said, I just didn't care for his manner or his attitude. He might be the best oncologist in the free world. I didn't feel comfortable enough to put my life in his hands.

Before he dismissed us, he told us that he was ordering a full body MRI and a series of bone scans for the next week and set an appointment for us to come back in two weeks.

We took the orders to the scheduler, right down the hall. The scheduler insisted that we couldn't get the tests done that soon. He told us that the first date he had available was sometime after the appointment the doctor had set up. That didn't make a lick of sense to me and I told him so. He then told me that he would set up the tests for the next week, like the doctor had ordered, but that we probably wouldn't get to do them as scheduled.

By now I felt like I was 97 and simply said, "Fine."

At least the doctor gave me a prescription for pain medication that would hopefully help my aching bones and allow me to get a little sleep at night. I was pretty dejected as we left the office and headed home—so much so that I declined Lisa's suggestion that we eat supper at Everybody's Pizza, opting instead for leftovers at home.

We stopped at the pharmacy to fill my prescription—again. Dr. Jamie came out to discuss our visit—again. We gave her the whole story and she mumbled that I needed to go to M.D. Anderson in Texas—again. Lisa insisted that we were fine in Atlanta—again.

Two days later, the scheduler called and said that we would have to wait two weeks to do the MRI and the nuclear bone scan and that we would have to, naturally, reschedule our office visit to go over the results until a week after the tests.

I honestly believed I could feel the cancer continue to grow in my body as I hung up the phone.

I waited patiently and kept my appointments at Emory University Hospital, which were all scheduled for late evening, something that seemed unusual to me. I suppose they have so many people who need treatment that they have to work around the clock almost—and let me say again, I am glad Emory is available in Atlanta. But the more I thought about things, the less I wanted to pursue treatment there.

I cancelled my appointment with the doctor at Emory and made one instead with Dr. Scott Miller. I wanted to hear what he had to say.

By the time I saw Dr. Miller, we had gotten the results of my tests. He told me that there were spots on my ribs and hips that indicated that my cancer had metastasized into my bones. My PSA was still doubling at a rapid rate. He agreed that we needed to seek treatment from an oncologist who specialized in advanced prostate disease and he agreed that the doctor we had seen at Emory was not the one we needed to treat my disease.

We talked about some options and we batted around the names of a couple of doctors in the area. I decided on one who practiced at Northside Cancer Center and we made an appointment to see him. Before saying our goodbyes, Dr. Miller advised me that my best course of action was hormone therapy. I had read about that on the internet. I had read about everything on the internet—but I listened as Dr. Miller explained how it worked.

"But aren't the side effects pretty drastic?" I asked.

That was the only time during our relationship that Scott Miller ever seemed to lose patience with me. "I'm not worried about side effects," he said. "I'm worried about you staying alive."

"Good point," I conceded. Then I asked him about the miracle diets that people had shared with me—like the one where you eat nothing but kale and pistachio nuts every day.

"None of those has ever been proved to work scientifically. And," he added, "there is a such thing as quality of life."

In essence he was saying what I had often thought. How long do you really want to live if you can't have a mess of fried catfish or a barbecue pork pig sandwich every once in a while?

Lisa and I went to visit the doctor that we had agreed upon on a Tuesday morning. I had read up on him, of course, and learned that he was one of the most widely respected advanced prostate practitioners in the Southeast. I was very despondent again by this time. I had little hope that this guy would offer any additional solutions. The people at Northside were very professional and realized that I was only 60. I appreciated their demeanor and efficiency. I even liked their waiting room. They actually had current magazines.

The nurse came in and went over my medical history and then the doctor came in. He was very succinct and matter-of-fact in his proclamations—and he began every sentence with, "So."

"So," he told me, "you have stage 4 metastatic prostate disease."

That hit me like a ton of bricks. I suspected that to be the case. I suppose that I knew it was and I had researched it on the internet, of course. I knew that the metastases, coupled with the rapidly increasing PSA numbers, didn't paint a very rosy picture, but still, hearing it spoken aloud by a doctor had quite an impact. I remember getting chill bumps and feeling nervous shivers running up and down my spine.

"So," he continued, "there is no cure but we can treat it as a chronic illness."

"What is the best way to treat it?" I asked.

"So," he replied, "the standard of care is to use Lupron, which is given as an injection every twelve weeks. Prostate cancer has been found to grow by consuming testosterone. The Lupron eliminates 95 percent of the testosterone in your body and slows down the spread of the cancer."

"For how long?" I asked.

"So," he replied, "we have patients we have been treating with Lupron for as long as ten years."

"What are the side effects?" was my next question.

"So," the doctor replied, "since the testosterone is destroyed, your sex drive will be basically eliminated and you will not be able to have an erection. You will have been chemically castrated. Also, over time your bone density will probably begin to deteriorate."

"Do you have any experimental treatments or options if this doesn't work?" was my last question for him.

"So," his answer was really a non-answer, but I am good at reading between the lines. "This is the standard care for stage 4 metastatic prostate disease."

"When can we begin the treatment?" I asked.

"So, we should begin right away. It will take a few days to get the treatment approved by your insurance, so I can order the injection today and we can set up an appointment for a couple of weeks."

I thanked him and asked him to order the injection and we left. I didn't want to go home, though. I wanted to do something to get my mind off the fact that I was convinced that I was dying. We got in the car and headed downtown. I wanted to visit the Georgia Aquarium. I had never been and in my mind I was certain that I wouldn't get another chance.

Lisa and I had a pleasant, if melancholy, time at the Aquarium. On the drove home, I pondered a lot of things in my mind and in my heart. As we pulled into the driveway, I looked at Lisa and said, just as matter-of-factly as the doctor had spoken, "So, we need to get an appointment at M.D. Anderson.

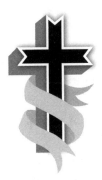

CHAPTER TWENTY THREE

God is good, all the time. All the time, God is good.

Late winter and early spring of 2012 was the darkest period of my life, so far, but God and God's people continued to pour blessing upon blessing upon me. Even on the days when I was as low as I thought I could possibly get, the encouragement and support and prayers of people I knew and people I did not know continued to lift me up.

The people of my community are amazing.

One day, Jean McCullough and some ladies from Conyers First United Methodist Church came by to bring me a beautiful handcrafted quilt. More than a hundred members of the church had autographed the quilt and written words of love and encouragement as well as promises from scripture on the quilt. Each word was like a gentle hug from God and I have spent many days and evenings in my recliner, wrapped up in that quilt, feeling the warm embrace of the people who bestowed it upon me.

On another day, Marshall Atha came by and brought me a similar quilt, which I equally treasure and use, from the congregation of the First Baptist Church in Covington. Marshall Atha is one of my favorite people in the whole world and I can't resist telling this story about him.

In 1995, I published my first book, Need Two. It was released in the fall and sold really, really well, especially in the weeks leading up to Christmas.

At that time, our kids were 10, 7, and 4—which meant that Santa Claus had needed lots and lots of help on Christmas Eve. Lisa and I had stayed up until 3 a.m. waiting for Santa to come. On Christmas Day we had made the rounds of parents and grandparents and aunts and uncles. Bedtime came early for us on Christmas night.

Shortly after midnight, my phone rang. I answered it, quite sleepily. I was surprised to hear Marshall on the other end of the line. "Darrell," he told me excitedly. "I got your book for Christmas. I just got through reading it and it was great. I laughed all day. It is the funniest book I ever read."

"I'm glad you liked my book, Marshall," I told him, "but it's after midnight. Couldn't you have waited until tomorrow to tell me?"

"But you don't understand," Marshall continued, as nonplussed as could be, "I haven't ever read but one other book and that was Black Beauty in the third grade. I just had to call and tell you how good it was."

That remains my favorite book review of my short and non-illustrious career as a writer.

The ladies from the local Catholic parish were prayer warriors as well, which shows to me that there are a lot more similarities in our Christian denominations than there are differences. They brought me a hand-knitted prayer shawl—in red and black. A couple of weeks later, they brought Lisa one, too. Even the Catholic Church in these parts realizes that God is a Bulldog.

Just kidding, y'all. My Tech friends were just as loyal and prayerful as my fellow Bulldogs and I appreciated their acts of mercy and kindness just as much.

I also received shawls and blankets and comforters from several other churches—too many to mention them all. The cards and letters and prayer-grams were amazing. I think every member of Newton Baptist Church in Covington and Salem Baptist Church in Stockbridge sent me at least two cards apiece. These were churches I had never attended, understand, and, in fact, couldn't have driven to them without asking directions.

The point I am trying to make is that during the darkest time of my journey, which for me was the month or so between the time I learned that the radiation had not worked and the time I walked into the M.D. Anderson Cancer Center for the first time. In that period, thousands of God's people were reaching out to me and letting me know that they were sharing His matchless love with me—just because. I had never been so touched in all my life, and if I live to be a hundred, or if I die tomorrow, I will carry to my grave the memories of all those compassionate people who offered me love and encouragement.

I will also carry with me the realization that there were too many times when I should have shown just as much compassion to my friends and acquaintances and failed to do so. I thought of John Kelly often during this period of time.

John Kelly was the father of one of my tennis players I coached at Heritage. Yes, I was once a girls' tennis coach, among many other things. Maria was John's daughter. She was an excellent student in my AP class and an excellent tennis player as well. Her dad was a little older than the other dads. I figured he was retired since he was the first to arrive at every match. He didn't seem to be encumbered by work, understand. I didn't know what he was retired from, but I thought he must be retired.

I always enjoyed chatting with him, and over the course of the season I learned that he was indeed retired—or at least semi-retired. He had spent an entire career in the United States Foreign Service, serving as Ambassador to Finland, which is where he found his beautiful wife, Maritza, and to Lebanon, where he had to wear a gun to work every day. He had also served as Deputy Secretary of State under James Baker in the Reagan administration. That's pretty high cotton. When I met John, he was doing a little consult work at Georgia Tech and he also worked as an expert of Middle East business affairs for anyone who needed expert advice.

You would never have guessed any of this if you had seen John at the tennis matches in his khakis and plaid shirt and floppy hat.

He told me a great story once about a dinner he had in the royal palace in Russia—although I think it was the Soviet Union at the time. I am not certain of all the dignitaries that were there, but I think Vice President George H.W. Bush and Secretary of State Jim Baker were two of them. That makes a better story, so I will assume they were the people he told me about.

The state dinner was being held in the great dining hall of the palace and, according to John, the place purely reeked of pretentiousness. He was given a leather-bound menu. Each gold-gilded page described the most elegant epicurean delights anyone could have imagined. John said that he spent thirty minutes pondering his choices. Finally it was time to order.

The waiter approached Vice President Bush and he pointed to the page containing the entrée he had decided upon. The waiter leaned close into Bush's ear and whispered something. Bush smiled and nodded. Next he approached the Secretary of State and the same thing happened. Baker pointed to an entrée, the waiter whispered in his ear and Baker smiled and nodded.

The waiter then approached John. John showed him the dish he had chosen and the waiter leaned in close and whispered, "We have chicken and potatoes."

John told me that he had the chicken and potatoes. And vodka. He said they had lots and lots of vodka.

Now I told you that to tell you this. About two years before I was diagnosed with cancer, John learned that he had AML—acute myeloid leukemia. I heard that he had cancer and intended to go and see him. For almost two years I intended to go and see him. I never did, however. I meant to. I wanted to. It would have benefitted me more than him because I loved talking with John and hearing his insight into the affairs of the world. I thought I knew a lot. John Kelly really did know a lot.

I ran into him at the grocery store every now and then and a few other places around town, and he always insisted he was fine. My friend from church, Keith Estes, who is one of those Tech people whose prayers so buoyed my own spirits, told me every Sunday, "You need to go and see John."

Every Sunday I told Keith, and myself, that I would. But I never did. When John died on September 15, 2011, I still hadn't been to visit and every time someone knocked on my door during my illness, I thought of John and realized how much my visit would have meant to him. And every time someone I thought I would have heard from didn't call or come by—I understood and knew they were somewhere meaning to.

But if I can offer this to you—if you ever hear of someone who needs a visit or a call or a note, visit or call or send a note. I now know, first-hand, how much visits and calls and cards mean to folks who are suffering and afraid and lonely.

Of course, I wasn't really lonely during this period because I had lots and lots of company at school. Teaching through this awful period was the best thing I could have done for myself. I'm not sure it was the best thing for my students but I hope they learned something. They each passed the all-powerful End of Course exams, so that was something. But I was slap worn out when I got home every day. I would head straight to my recliner and immediately fall asleep.

Day after day, my friend Gary, himself a retired teacher, would come by to keep me company. Sometimes he would sit and talk; sometimes he would watch TV while I slept. Sometimes he would just sit. I always appreciated his presence. I never told him so, I don't think—or at least not often enough.

I often thought during this period about Buddy Neel, who reminded me that a heavy load is made lighter if there are a lot of people to share the lifting. I had so many people to help me share the lifting. For every person I have mentioned by name there were dozens of people I should mention. Many of them were people I knew only through Facebook. Let me tell you something—Facebook friends can be quite a community.

I have a large number of Facebook friends—about 3,500 and growing, actually. Many are my real-life friends, of course. Many are long-lost high school classmates with whom I have lost touch over the years—not to mention decades. Many are former students and many are my readers whom I have never met in person. Once Buddy convinced me to share my story, I shared with everybody. I told strangers in the grocery store. I wrote about it in my columns. And I posted on Facebook. I posted about my good days and my bad days and got a world of encouragement on both. When I felt like I needed prayers, I asked for them.

Does not the Bible say "Ask and ye shall receive?" When I asked my Facebook friends for prayer, I got prayers in droves. Prayers work. I could feel them working. I ain't just whistling Dixie, understand, I am testifying to what I know. My Facebook friends even seemed to sense when I needed funds for tests or treatments or travel. Every time my bank account neared zero, my Facebook friends seem to light up my website with book orders.

God seemed to know what I needed, too. He knew that I needed to stay busy in February so that I wouldn't have to sit around thinking about my problems. I had a fairly busy December and didn't schedule any appearances to speak of in January. By the end of the month, my cupboard was not only bare, the moths were actually begging for table scraps, figuratively speaking, of course. God put me on the road in February, and the people to whom I spoke were generous beyond measure, in many ways.

As the great Methodist preacher and Wesley scholar John Beyers is wont to say, they offered me heartbeats of love in negotiable form— and love and support and encouragement and prayers. They gave me lots and lots of prayers. Are you beginning to understand how much importance I place in the power of prayer?

One of the first talks I made in the new year was at a Friends of the Library benefit in the Newton County Public Library in Covington. I stayed away from that library for a long time because I checked out Henry Aaron, RF from there when I was a teenager and never returned it. I was afraid the statute of limitations on overdue books had not expired and thought I might owe them $3 million dollars or something.

We had a big crowd at that meeting and I was happy to be back on my feet, talking to people who weren't mandated by a compulsory attendance law to be there. Halfway through my spiel I noticed that my good friend, Wheeler Davidson, looked a little pale. Actually, he looked real pale. In fact, he looked awful. He got up and left the room. I wasn't sure what I should do so I just kept talking. A moment later he came back into the room and summoned his bride, Ginny.

Wheeler was having a heart attack, right in the middle of my speech. Ever the Southern gentleman, he didn't interrupt or cause a commotion, he just quietly left the room and had his wife drive him to the local hospital. Amazing.

But, then again, Wheeler Davidson is an amazing human being. I first met him when I was teaching and coaching football and girls' basketball at Clarkston High School in the early 1980s. Go Goats!

Wheeler, who hails from Lithonia and is a proud graduate of North Georgia College, was a teacher in the history department and we ate lunch together most days surrounded by the most liberal ladies, politically, that you could ever imagine. I was a recent convert myself, and Wheeler and I defended Ronald Reagan every day. We felt like the last great bastion of conservatism in DeKalb County and became fast friends. We became even faster friends when I realized that he was as big a Georgia football fan as I am.

Every Friday in the fall, Wheeler would make a point of finding me to talk about the next day's game and tell me that he was almost ready for his tailgate. "I've done everything but go by Greene's" he would say. Greene's is a famous package store in the Atlanta area, in case you aren't from around here.

Fast-forward 25 years and I crossed Wheeler's path again when my dear friends Martha and Bob Mann invited me to join their tailgate group for a Georgia game. I came to find out that Wheeler was the self-appointed, non-elected and can't-be-fired Chairman of the Oak Tree Tailgate gang. He and his group had been tailgating in the same spot for more than two decades, and Lisa and I were honored when they invited us to be a part of the group. That was ten years ago and now Wheeler and the other "oaks" are practically family. And here I was giving the Chairman Emeritus a heart attack during my first outing after my self-imposed sabbatical. I was ashamed of myself.

Wheeler is a tough old bird, however. The good people at Emory took wonderful care of him and he made a remarkable recovery. As the 2012 football season approaches, Wheeler is ready to run the table one more time and plans to attend every game, home and away, that the Bulldogs play.

I hope I can do that when I'm 81. Heck, I hope I can do that when I am 61.

My other engagements were less dramatic, but I was heartened everywhere I went by the fact that most of the people I encountered were aware of my situation and told me that they had been praying for me for a long time. I am constantly relating these stories of intercessory prayer on my behalf so that everyone who reads this book will be reminded of the words handed down by God, through the scriptures.

"Do not be anxious about anything, but in everything,
by prayer and petition, with thanksgiving, present
your requests to God." Philippians 4:6 NIV

"First of all, then, I urge that supplications, prayers,
intercessions, and thanksgivings be made for all people.
" I Timothy 2:1 ESV

"Likewise the Spirit helps us in our weakness. For we do not know
what to pray for as we ought, but the Spirit himself intercedes for
us with groanings too deep for words. And he who searches hearts
knows what is the mind of the Spirit, because the Spirit intercedes
for the saints according to the will of God." Romans 8: 26-27. ESV

"Therefore, confess your sins to one another and pray for one
another, that you may be healed. The prayer of a righteous person
has great power as it is working." James 5: 16 ESV

"Whatever you ask in my name, this I will do,
that the Father may be glorified in the Son." John 14:13 ESV

Prayer works. How do I know? The Bible tells me so—and I have experienced the power of prayer first hand. My body did not begin to miraculously heal immediately, but my soul did. As more and more people confirmed to me that they were claiming healing on my behalf, in the name of Christ Jesus, my fears began to subside. When I lay down at night and turned to God in prayer, my supplications were no longer limited to the "groaning too deep for words" that Paul wrote about in his letter to the Romans. I could actually talk to God. I could share my heart with him. I could confess my sins and let God know that I had sincerely repented of them. I could carry on a conversation with God.

Think about that! We have the capacity, as human beings, to carry on a conversation with God Almighty. In my Forrest Gump-like existence, I have had the opportunity to talk to some pretty impressive people. I have spoken with Bear Bryant, Adolph Rupp, Johnny Cash, George Bush, Barbara Dooley—I used to receive calls from Lester Maddox every Saturday morning.

But every day, whenever the notion strikes me, I can pause and have a conversation with God. I love Barbara Dooley, but talking to her doesn't compare with talking to the Creator of the universe and the Supreme Judge of the World.

Prayers for healing were being answered. I was being healed—from the inside out. God was addressing my most crucial infirmity first—my immortal soul.

Please do not hear something I am not saying. I didn't lose my fears overnight and from time to time I still had desperate moments of doubt, but I was moving toward that perfect peace that only comes from being one with the Lord.

Toward the middle of February, during my school's winter break, Lisa and I headed out on a memorable road trip to Florida. Our first stop was Jacksonville to visit with Terri and Steve Cooper and to speak at their church. Terri and I were kindred spirits during high school and college. Ours was a friendship that defies explanation.

We were never boyfriend and girlfriend—exactly—but we were also closer than just good friends. It's complicated.

I rarely see Terri these days, but no matter how long we go between visits—and sometimes it has been years—we can just pick up where we left off. Terri took us out to Jacksonville Beach and patiently drove up and down the strip, helping me look for an old boarding house where my family always stayed on vacation back in the 1950s. We found it, too. Then climbed the Red Cross tower and visited the Mayo Clinic.

I was impressed by Mayo and gathered all the information they had, but after talking with the people there realized that they didn't have any programs for my particular situation that weren't available in Atlanta.

After speaking to a very receptive group at Terri and Steve's church we headed across the state the following morning to the heart of the Redneck Riviera—Panama City Beach, to speak to the Emerald Coast Bulldog Club. This was an entirely different kind of group, but I reconnected with an old friend from college, Darryl Jones, and made some new best friends as well—and picked up a few more prayer warriors.

My busy month continued as the following week I had two engagements in Athens and had the great honor of bringing the Ash Wednesday message at the Conyers First United Methodist Church. That was a big, big deal for me—to be invited to stand in the pulpit of that great church with John Beyers seated beside me—speaking not of good times in Porterdale or Georgia football, but of the love and sacrifice of God's son who died for my personal sins.

I could sense a change in the direction of my life that day. I didn't know where that turn was going to take me, but I was willing to let Jesus take control and was bound to follow wherever He led.

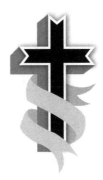

CHAPTER TWENTY FOUR

I kept up my hectic speaking schedule throughout February. I am sure a lot of people felt like I must have been faking the whole cancer thing because I was teaching school every day and writing three columns a week and traveling all over the Southeast—or so it seemed—talking to anyone who would give me an invitation and listen to me. I heard the same thing over and over and over: "You look great!"

I realized that what they meant was, "You look great for someone suffering from stage 4 cancer who has one foot in the grave and the other on a banana peel." I overlooked that, however, and just said thank you because, in reality, it made me feel really good to hear it.

Actually, getting out amongst folks helped keep me going. I've known for a long time that it is better to wear out than rust out. My mama and daddy instilled in me a great work ethic—despite what my lovely wife, Lisa, might have you believe. I never have believed in just sitting around on my duff. Besides, what good would that have done? I would have had way too much time to think negative thoughts—so, yes, I was worn out physically, but I wouldn't do it any differently if I had it to do over.

And everywhere I went I picked up more and more prayer warriors and could feel the power of each one.

Toward the end of February, I had the great honor of being asked by Camille Braswell to serve as Honorary Chairperson of the Boule' on Bourbon Cancer Benefit at the Classic Center in Athens. You talk about putting on the dog! They had turned the Foundry into New Orleans. They had streetlights and balconies and beads, raw oysters and shrimp and grits, and some of the best music I have ever heard. They had everything Bourbon Street has except strippers. At least, if they had those, I didn't see them. The whole shindig was to raise money for the Light up the Night campaign to raise money for cancer research.

Lisa and I got to dress up and be in the spotlight while the very crème of Athens society danced the night away. We even got to stay overnight at one of those fancy downtown hotels. My only regret was that the benefit was only seven months after my surgery instead of eight. Go back and reread if you need to. I made a little speech and promised the crowd that I would be back the following year to celebrate a full recovery. I hope they get to hold me to it.

I spoke at all sorts of other functions, too. I addressed the Georgia Association of Education Leaders. Now that was fun! I got to stand before principals and school superintendents, including my own, on Super Bowl Sunday—which is why I was asked to pinch hit for the governor in the first place—and tease the leadership of Georgia schools about all the things the federal and state governments are making us do wrong in education. They all laughed because they knew every word I said was true.

I spoke to retired educators and church groups and Rotary Clubs and old lady sewing circles. It was fun. I love to show off, and I hate to say it, but having cancer is apparently good for book sales. Sometimes I would get invited to places I had already been before and would have a really hard time remembering which stories I had told before. It didn't matter so much at the senior citizen dinners because if I couldn't remember, they certainly couldn't, but some of the younger set had better memories. Of course, sometimes, if I left out a certain story, folks would call for it from the audience.

Take the story about the 2007 Georgia-Florida football game, for instance. Unlike most of what I tell, this one is 100 percent true. Georgia started off struggling that year, and when it came time to make the annual trip to the World's Largest Outdoor Cocktail Party at the end of October, a lot of Georgia fans had dumped their tickets on eBay, StubHub and the like. So, when I got to my seats at the game, there were Florida fans all around me, and it irritated me because I spend a lot of money to keep from having to sit among the riffraff.

Every year I sit at the Georgia-Florida game with my buddy, Chris Timmerman. Chris was raised at North Myrtle Beach, and his daddy, Dick, and I go way back. Dick Timmerman is one of the best people I know and would give me the shirt off his back if I needed it. Chris was a little snot-nosed gym rat hanging around his daddy's recreation department when I first met him. Now he is a grown man and married with kids of his own. He and his beautiful bride, Dyana, live in Jacksonville, Fla. Chris and I watch dozens of football and basketball games and golf matches together every year. He sits on his couch in Florida and I sit in my chair in Conyers and we text back and forth throughout whatever contest it is we are watching. But once a year we get to sit beside one another at a game.

Now I told you all that to tell you this. Chris was with me as we walked up to our seats and saw all those Gators where I was going to have to sit. I turned to him and said, "Whatever happens, don't let me spend the night in the Jacksonville jail."

There was orange and blue on my right and orange and blue on my left and orange and blue behind me. There were two empty seats in front of me. I sat down and prayed, "God, please don't let there be Florida fans sitting there, too."

God didn't answer that one. Just before kickoff, a Florida student came up and sat down. Typical Gator. Mullet. Jean shorts. Ugly. Bad teeth. Pimples. And her date looked worse than she did.

The guy had one of those big foam fingers that proclaim, "We're No. 1," and he sat it down under his seat and turned right toward me and did the Gator Chomp right in my face. Scrunched up his face. Showed me his bad teeth. Right in my face.

Believe it or not, I ignored him. We kicked off to Florida, and on the first play from scrimmage, quarterback Tim Tebow got a first down and my Florida friend turned around and did that Gator Chomp right in my face again. My blood was boiling.

Florida got another first down and he did it again. This time I had had all I could take.

I tapped the guy on the shoulder and said, "Friend, I am going to give you some good advice. Now you can take it or leave it. It's a free country. But it is good advice.

"Now, you can stand up and cheer for your team and holler hurrah for Florida and do anything you want to do, but if you do that Gator Chomp in my face one more time, you and your friends will come to this game every year for the next fifty years and every conversation you have will begin with, 'Remember that time that sixty-year-old man whipped your ass at the Georgia-Florida game?'"

Well, that got off with him. He turned around and on the next play, Tebow threw an interception. I celebrated by pounding my new buddy on the back—hard—and screaming, "How 'bout them Dawgs!" right in his ear. He knew I was at the game, understand.

Two plays later, UGA's tailback, Knowshon Mareno, scored a touchdown and I was pounding and screaming some more. Then the dangdest thing happened. Georgia coach, Mark Richt, sent the entire Bulldog team into the end zone to celebrate. That's a little bit illegal in case you aren't a big football fan.

Chris tapped me on the shoulder and said, "Did you see what they just did?"

I just grinned stupidly and nodded. I was having too much fun celebrating on the Florida guy's back to respond. Chris said, "Georgia is fixing to kick off from the seven yard line! Have you ever seen anything like this?"

I was talking to Chris but I was right in the Gator's ear and said, "I ain't never seen anything like this."

Chris said, "How long have you been coming to these games?

I said, "I have been to every Georgia-Florida game since 1966, except for the three years I was in prison for killing that guy at the 1980 game."

The Florida fan whispered something to his date, then they left and we didn't see them anymore. We did win the game, however.

Folks seem to like to hear that story and the closer to Athens I get, the more they seem to like it. I told it at Terri Cooper's church in

Jacksonville, however, and didn't even draw a snicker. I didn't say "ass," either. Oh, well. No accounting for taste.

All of my stories are rooted in truth, although there may be a bit of exaggeration here and there. My good friend and mentor, Uncle Jack Bowden, taught me that you should never let the truth stand in the way of a good story.

Speaking of good stories, here's another favorite. This one came about a couple of Februaries ago. It was a cold, wet, rainy afternoon—just a nasty day. We had been to Sunday school and church, and I was sitting in front of a nice warm fire watching Duke play basketball on television after dinner.

Lisa came in and said, "Put on your coat. I want you to go with me to Lowe's to buy some light bulbs."

What I wanted to say was, "Why do you need me to go with you to buy light bulbs? They aren't heavy. You can carry them."

But since Lisa controls 70 percent of the money and 100 percent of the sex in my life, what I actually said was, "Yes, dear."

We got to Lowe's and found the light bulbs. It was easy. They were right under a sign marked "Illuminare." We picked out what she needed and I foolishly headed toward the register. I thought I could get home for the last few minutes of the game.

"Wait a minute," Lisa said, followed by, "as long as we are here..."

As soon as I heard, "As long as we are here," I knew I was in trouble. Expensive trouble.

"What?" I asked, knowing full well that it didn't matter.

"As long as we're here, we might as well look at the ovens."

"The ovens!" I thought. I sure didn't see that one coming. We already had a good oven. We got it when we built our house, twenty-eight years ago. It cooked great food.

What I said, though, was, "Yes, dear." Hey, operation or not, I still needed money.

They had ovens at Lowe's and we found one that I thought was perfect. It was a 28-inch double oven that was pretty much like the one we had at home, except 28 years newer. It was on sale, too—for $999.99. I figured that it would last at least as long as I would and got ready to write the man a check.

You'd think I'd know better after thirty years. Lisa said, "We aren't going to buy the first oven we come across."

I said, "Lisa, we didn't just come across this oven. We left the warm fireplace and went out into the cold rain looking for it!"

"Nope," she said. "We're going over to see what they have at Sears."

What they had at Sears was a Kenmore 28-inch double oven exactly like the one we had at home—same controls, same wiring, same everything—and it was on sale for $850. "We'll take it," I told the man, and started writing out the check before he decided to take the sale price off.

The Sears man pretended to write up the sale, but just before he got to the part where he started trying to sell me a long-term warranty—you know, as soon as he'd told me how durable the appliance was—he said, "Before we do this, let me show you what we have over here."

If the Sears man ever tells your wife, "Let me show you what we have over here," just go ahead and hand him your credit cards, your checkbook and all your cash. You are fixing to let go of some jack.

What he had "over here" was a 30-inch stainless steel double convection oven—with every kind of bell and whistle and button and bow you can imagine. It cost $3,600. My car didn't cost $3,600. But this oven was on sale—for half price, $1,800.

"We are going to save almost $2,000," Lisa exclaimed.

That's women's math. In men's math, we were going to spend an extra $950. Plus tax. But in women's math, we were going to save $1,800 by buying a $3,600 oven instead of an $850 one. I paid the man and loaded up the oven and drove home through the rain. When we got home the ball game was over.

When we got home is when I also realized that it doesn't matter what you cut out or how hard you try, you can't put a 30-inch oven in a 28-inch cabinet. We were at a cabinet shop Monday afternoon, picking out new counters. We just had to have granite countertops. I could have bought Stone Mountain for what I paid for those countertops.

We got the oven and the countertops and the cabinets installed, and the floors looked so bad next to the new furnishings that we had to have the floor replaced. And then the paint was dull, so we had to paint—and get new light fixtures. I also learned that you can't have an almond-colored refrigerator in the same kitchen with a stainless steel oven.

We got the whole kitchen redone and then we had to do something about the windows. My mama had curtains in her house her whole life. We don't have curtains in our house anymore. We have window treatments. My buddy asked me, "What's the difference between curtains and window treatments?"

I said, "As near as I can figure, about $1,200."

But we got that kitchen looking good. Of course, it's right next to the dining room and the dining room is next to the kitchen, so they both had to be redone.

If you ever want to see a $50,000 light bulb, drop by my house and I'll show you one. Sixty-seven more payments and that bad boy is all mine.

Those are the sort of stories I sometimes tell, depending on the audience, of course. Usually I end with an inspirational moment, maybe a poem—I like reciting poetry—or maybe a short testimony, if I am at a church. Throughout the winter and spring of 2012, my talks began to change a right smart, as the folks I worked with in the mill used to say. I still tried to make people laugh and I still told stories about my kids and growing up in Porterdale, and some of the stories were even true, but I began to feel an urge to cut down a bit on the stories and expand the testimony.

God was working on me. He had really gotten my attention when I started reading those statistics on the internet. Twelve to eighteen months might seem like an awfully long jail sentence, but it doesn't seem very long at all when it refers to the average life expectancy of 80 percent of the men in my specific situation. I started looking for opportunities to speak my piece at churches. I even put out a call on Facebook for folks who wanted to hear my story.

One of the first to answer that all-call was my lifetime friend, Todd Hilton, pastor of the Mansfield United Methodist Church.

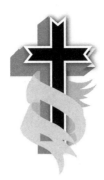

CHAPTER TWENTY FIVE

Todd Hilton's people and I go back a long way. His grandmother, Iris Standard, and my mother worked together in the weave shop of the Osprey Mill for a long, long time, and were very close friends. Mrs. Iris was a lay speaker in the Methodist church and was the first woman preacher I knew anything about. Every year she would deliver the Easter morning sunrise service at the Julia A. Porter Methodist Church.

I loved hearing her preach. She didn't stand behind the pulpit. She stood right up in front of the altar rail and she used illustrations about ballplayers, like Lou Gehrig, and things I could relate to, even as a small boy. I can close my eyes and still see her standing there and I can still hear her voice talking about Jesus and Simon Peter from the Salem Road abridged translation of the Bible.

From John:21:

"Peter do you love me?"
"Lord you know I love you!"
"Feed my lambs."
"Peter, do you love me?"
"Yes, Lord. You know I do!"
"Tend my sheep."
"Peter, do you love me?"
"Lord, why do you keep asking me this.
You know I love you more than anything."
"Take care of my sheep."

I will always remember hearing Iris Standard proclaiming the word of God and will always cherish that memory.

When I was a small boy, I used to ride to sunrise service with my next-door neighbor, Miss Mae Hardman. Miss Mae didn't drive for a long time and Mrs. Annie Lee Day, the nurse you met in one of the earlier chapters of this book, would pick us up. We would go to the cemetery first and put flowers on the grave of Mrs. Annie's late husband.

By the time Mrs. Annie was no longer able to drive very well, Miss Mae had taken up driving and bought a car of her own. She would do the driving on Easter until I turned sixteen and I could drive. Then I would drive them both. The last Easter that Mrs. Annie was alive, and maybe the last Easter that Mrs. Iris preached at sunrise service, I was in the Newton County hospital being diagnosed for a mysterious stomach ailment that to this day hasn't cleared up. I got one of my friends to leave a car and a set of clothes in the hospital parking lot, and right after the nurse made her morning rounds, I climbed out the window of my room—luckily the hospital only had one floor back then—and took Mrs. Annie Lee Day and Miss Mae Hardman to sunrise service at Porterdale. I snuck back in the window before anyone knew I was gone.

Mrs. Iris would be so proud if she knew that her grandson, Todd, has made a preacher and is doing a grand job, breathing new life into that famous old country church in Mansfield.

Todd invited me to come and speak at a Sunday night service, just a few days before my first trip to M.D. Anderson.

I know. I know. I haven't said too much about M.D. Anderson yet. But like Gene Talmadge said to the guy in the tree that shouted, "Tell us about the crooked politicians in Washington," I'm a comin' to that!

I didn't know what to expect when I showed up in Mansfield that night. I had spoken at thousands of events and hundreds of churches, but for some reason this felt different. I believed that God was sending me to Mansfield for a different purpose than to entertain and inspire. When I walked into the church and saw the crowd gathered there, I knew immediately that God had indeed sent me to Mansfield for a different purpose. He sent me there to receive a blessing, not to bestow one.

I couldn't believe how many people were gathered there and I couldn't believe who some of the folks were. Some of my Facebook friends had traveled a hundred miles to hear me just because they had read the post that I would be there. Scotty Kimble was in the house and I hadn't seen Scotty more than a handful of times since I coached him in middle school football and basketball.

Doug and Carol Doster, beloved members of Julia A. Porter, were there. I love Doug and Carol, even if Doug is an unrepentant Georgia Tech fan. Doug is simply good people and so is Carol. I hope Doug never goes into stand-up because I don't need the competition in our area. One night at an adult Sunday school party, Gayle Norton was in charge of the entertainment and she had some of the couples in attendance play her version of the Newlywed Game. She asked the question, "What hymn best represents your spouse's opinion of your wedding night?" Doug answered, "How Great Thou Art!"

I was shocked to see that Jerry Aldridge and Mrs. A were there. Mrs. A—aka Lee Aldridge—was my high school biology teacher. If ever a teacher was cool, Mrs. A was cool. She talked in a language high school students could understand. At least once a day, I exclaim in my own classroom, "Well, 'Hark, a lark!' in tribute to her. She adopted a lot of us and we could think of no higher honor to bestow upon her than rolling her yard as often as possible, tossing every roll of paper into the trees with pure unadulterated love.

Of course, she always made us come over and clean it up the next day, but that just gave us more time to be around her.

I'll bet Lee Aldridge has visited more hospital rooms and attended more weddings than any other person in the Northeast Georgia Piedmont. When my mama was on her deathbed, Mrs. A came to see her and brought her a ceramic angel that I still treasure to this day.

Mama died a few days before Christmas. On the day before Christmas Eve, for no particular reason, as Forrest Gump might say, Mrs. A came to my house and brought me a beautifully illustrated copy of 'Twas the Night Before Christmas. The next year she did the same thing, and the next and the next and the next.

She has given me more copies and versions of that little book than you can imagine exist. I have the Redneck Night Before Christmas and the Teacher's Night Before Christmas and the Cajun Night Before Christmas, as well as pop-up versions, miniature versions, you name it and Mrs. A has brought it to my backdoor at Christmas time. On Christmas Eve, we always pick out a different version to sit on the hearth and read.

You wouldn't believe how much my kids began to look forward to the visit from "The Christmas Book Lady."

Every year she sees me and every year she says, "The books are over. I just can't find any editions you don't have." Every year, a few days before Christmas, I get a text from one of the kids, "She came and brought another book!"

I take one thing back, though. With apologies to Forrest, she doesn't do it for no particular reason. She does it because she loves me and I love her.

Her husband, Jerry, and I have a completely different bond: the Boy Scouts of America. When I made Eagle Scout, Jerry arranged for the Bibb to send me to Philmont Scout Ranch near Cimarron, New Mexico, with a crew of Scouts that Jerry had put together and attached to a larger contingent from the Atlanta Area Council. I learned more about self-reliance and camping and backpacking and leadership on that trip than I had learned in the previous sixteen years of my life—and had more fun.

Five years later, Jerry and I went back to Philmont together. This time I was a leader, too, and would continue going back to Philmont until I got married and Lisa made me quit being a Boy Scout. Jerry never did quit and has helped produce more than fifty Eagle Scouts and has made a huge difference in the lives of thousands of boys.

I love Jerry, too.

As I sat there in Mansfield United Methodist Church waiting my turn to speak, I gazed at the faces of more and more people, amazed that they would all give up their Sunday evening to travel down to Mansfield to support me and hear what I had to say. I was so empowered by God's love expressed by these good people. And then I saw Margaret.

Margaret would be Margaret Autry, Stump's wife. Stump would be Jeff Autry, the best friend I ever had in my entire life.

How can I explain the relationship I developed with the Autry family? I cannot. Not really. Words cannot adequately describe how two families can so completely intertwine as to become one, but that's how things worked out with the Autrys and the Huckabys.

When Greg, Jeff and Margaret's middle son, was in the sixth grade, he tried out for my Cousins Middle School football team. I had a no-cut policy but I didn't have a policy against kids quitting and I tried my best to run Greg off—not because I didn't like him, but because he was so little. And he wasn't like the other little kids that just wanted to be on the team for the glory of belonging and were willing to hang back out of the way when the rough drills began. Greg wanted to play, and he kept lining himself up against the biggest and strongest kids in all the contact drills. I really did think he would get himself killed.

I noticed the first week of practice that a big delivery truck drove up to the end of the parking lot. A man with a belly as big as my daddy's—and as big as mine is now—climbed on the top of the truck to watch practice. I thought at first that it was probably a spy from our cross-town rivals, Sharp Middle School. But one day after practice, as I was walking off the field, the guy climbed down off the truck and came up and introduced himself.

"I'm Jeff Autry," he said. "This is our business," he added, pointing to the truck. "Holifield sausage. We make it and I sell it. I'm the little boy's daddy—Greg's daddy." Then he said, "If we can ever help you in any way, you just let me know." Almost as an afterthought he added, "I would never tell you how to coach, but don't be afraid to let Greg hit. If he gets hurts, we got good insurance."

After that, I let Greg hit anybody he wanted to line up against. It was apparent that he wasn't going to give up, so I kept him on the team. I found out that he was really smart and understood the game. I put him at flanker, where all the kids that were too small for football played, but I also put him in the rotation sometimes if the play was going to be run away from him because I knew he would get the right play delivered to our quarterback.

I still remember how proud Greg was the day I gave out the game uniforms. The only pair that would fit him had grass stains all over them, but it was middle school football. It was what it was and the small kid who ran in the plays sometimes got the grass-stained pants.

I admonished the entire team that whatever they did, they were not to bleach their white football pants. The synthetic fiber the pants were made of wouldn't pass the Clorox test. The day before the first game of the season, Greg came up in tears—and with his pants in sparkling white threads.

"Your mama bleached those pants, boy!" I growled. "Why didn't you tell her not to bleach them pants?"

"She didn't," Greg insisted. "I told her not to. She swears she didn't bleach them."

It was fifteen years before Margaret Autry would admit that she just couldn't let her little boy go out on that football field with grass-stained pants and that she had, indeed, bleached the tar out of them.

The first game of that year, we were playing Carver Middle School in Monroe. The game was a defensive classic, which in middle school football talk means that neither team's offense was good enough to move the ball. We were down to the final minutes and we had the ball near midfield. It was now or never. We were going to use the whole halfback pass—shades of Appleby to Washington!

Greg swears that he didn't do it, but I am absolutely certain that he sent our left halfback to right halfback, the position I intended for him to play. All I know is that when our team broke the huddle and lined up in our old-fashioned T-formation, Greg was at left half and was about to throw the ball.

I had already used up my timeouts so there was nothing to do but let nature take its course. Our quarterback, Greg Cowan, made a perfect pitch to Greg Autry, who looked like a Pee Wee Leaguer coming around the end. Just before being buried under the entire Carver team, Greg pulled up and threw a perfect spiral to our split-end, Michael Smith, racing down the right sideline for the winning touchdown.

When the season was over, I gave Greg a football and told him to throw it until the cows came home—and to grow four inches and gain thirty pounds. I anointed him quarterback for the next season. He did all three and led the Cousins Rams to the Middle Georgia Junior High Athletic League Championship. That was a big deal, too, because the Middle Georgia League covered several counties— from Fayetteville to Greensboro—and had a membership of about twenty-six teams.

The championship game was cakewalk, but the semi-finals against Dan Gabriel's undefeated Morgan County Bulldogs was an all-out nuclear war. We played in the rain in Madison on a Monday night. The game was back and forth all night, but with less than two minutes left in the game, Morgan County scored to go up by five. It was something like 27-20.

It had been drizzling all night and now the rain had picked up. The field and the ball were going to be wet. I didn't care. I grabbed our center, Jeff Smalley—whose dad, Jack, had played for Bear Bryant at Alabama—and literally picked him up off his feet. I looked him right in the eye and said, "Boy, can you snap a wet ball."

He looked me square in the eye and said, "Yes, sir," without so much as a waver in his voice.

Then I grabbed Greg's arm and told him to get in the single wing, which means he would become a blocking back with direct snaps to our halfbacks—kind of like the "new-fangled" Wildcat formation teams run today, but not exactly. I told him to send running back, Vincent Price, left and our other running back, Jarvis Andrews, right.

Jeff made perfect snaps on every play. Greg—and the rest of the team—blocked liked Bronco Nagurski and we went through Morgan County like a dose of salts through a widow woman. Five plays later and we had scored, cutting our deficit to 27-26. I called a timeout to talk about the extra point, which would win or lose the game for us.

Greg looked like the perfect picture of the quarterback as he calmly trotted over. He had a confident gleam in his bright blue eyes. His blonde hair was curling out from under his helmet. "What's it going to be, Greg?" I asked him. "28? 49? Maybe a bootleg? You want to throw the tight-end dump?"

He looked at me and said, "I'm not crazy. You're the coach. You pick the play."

I told him to run sweep left and sent him back out on the field. At the last minute I screamed, "Sweep right!" He just looked over his shoulder and winked at me. He snapped the ball to Jarvis Andrews, who headed for the pylon with three Bulldogs in hot pursuit. Jarvis dove for the flag—and landed in the end zone, just inside the pylon. We had won, 28-27.

I looked back over my shoulder and Jeff Autry was halfway up a light standard, holding on for dear life.

That was a magical year. We won our league in football and basketball, and over the course of that season, Jeff Autry became closer to me than any friend I had ever had—or would ever have. And poor Margaret. God had already blessed her with a husband and three sons, and now she had adopted another male member of the family.

I was single at the time and would go by my mama's house for supper after practice every evening. Then I would go to the Autry's to see Jeff. Luckily for me, they ate about 40 minutes later than we did and I would always get to their house just as Margaret was putting supper in the table. Every night she would invite me to eat and I couldn't bring myself to hurt her feelings by turning her down.

After supper, Jeff and I would usually go out and drink coffee at Jim Stalvey's restaurant at the Crest Hotel in Covington. We would talk about football and life and selling sausage. Jeff would tell me about growing up at the Jolly Home in Conyers, which at that time was an orphanage, and playing ball with my future father-in-law and Tommy Lee McCurty and other Rockdale County legends. I would tell him about my dreams of one day becoming a writer and having people read my books and newspaper columns.

Most people laughed when I told them I wanted to do that. Jeff didn't laugh. He just told me to dedicate the first book to him. When Need Two was released, the dedication page read "For Stump." He wasn't alive to see it, though. His life had been cut short by a sudden heart attack a couple of years earlier.

By then our families' lives had become permanently intertwined, even though I don't see Margaret or Greg or her other two sons, Jeff and Matt, nearly often enough. I know, however, that if I ever needed anything in the world, I could call on any of them and they would never let me down.

When I saw Margaret sitting in that congregation, tears flowed down my face and I knew that I could not give my regular spiel that night. I was honored to stand in the pulpit of that church and share with the many, many friends who had gathered there what God was doing in my spiritual life. I was about to leave for my first trip to M.D. Anderson in just a few days and I was scared and hurting and weary, but I had been having daily and nightly talks with Jesus and we had reached an understanding. He would do what he wanted to do with my life and I would try to do what he wanted me to do with it, too. But, as I told that wonderful group of people that night, "No matter what condition my body is in, all is well with my soul."

After my message, everyone there gathered around me and I was anointed with prayer. Then Todd Hilton passed the plate and collected a love offering to help with my travel to Houston. He handed me exactly $360. That was the same amount of money Lisa and I had saved by changing hotels on our honeymoon. It was the exact amount of money our plane fare home from New Orleans had been. When we drove to Houston and back on that first M.D. Anderson run we spent $360 on gas and lodging.

Just another God-incident.

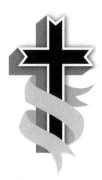

CHAPTER TWENTY SIX

OK. It is time to talk about the University of Texas M.D. Anderson Cancer Center, which I believe is the finest cancer treatment facility in the world. I admit that I haven't been to every cancer treatment facility in the world, but I cannot imagine there being a better one. I had never heard of M.D. Anderson until I heard my daughter, Jamie Leigh, mention it in the pharmacy one day.

I began to do a bit of investigation myself. I read everything I could on the internet—there I go, getting on the internet again!—and I talked to a few people who had been treated there. My friend Fred Harwell made a comment on every Facebook post I made, demanding that I go to Houston. Fred never was the subtle type. Once he said, and I quote, "What's the matter with you? Do you want to die? GO TO M.D. ANDERSON."

I don't think Fred believes that cancer can be treated anywhere else.

To tell the truth, I had been trying to get an appointment in Texas since the day we came back from the doctor who first told me, "So, you have Stage 4 metastasized prostate disease." I quickly learned that, while the facility tries to be as accessible as possible, there are a lot of people who want to be treated at the finest place on the planet. It's not as easy as calling up and saying I'd like to drop in next Tuesday.

I contacted them by phone and they told me that I would need to send all of my records from all of my doctors, as well as all of my test results, since I first started having problems. They needed all of that information so that they could evaluate my case and assign my case to the doctors best suited to deal with me. That made sense.

There was just one thing. Isn't there always just one thing? I had seen more than two dozen doctors in more than a dozen places and had had tests run in ten different places. That's a lot of records to be compiled, even when you have someone as efficient and medically aware as my lovely wife.

There were other considerations, too. Houston, Texas, is a long way from Conyers, Georgia. Plus there is that thing about the unknown. I have always boasted, especially to my kids, that I am not afraid of anything or anybody. My friend, Blake Craft, used to tell me the only thing he was afraid of was to get to heaven and hear Jesus say, "You've been tried in the balance and found wanting." I was afraid of that, but I am also a little uncomfortable with the unknown and things I cannot control. Keep that statement in the back of your mind for future reference.

M.D. Anderson Cancer Center was an unknown entity and I was a bit wary of turning my future over to them, even though I do have a great respect for the state of Texas and Texans in general. But to make Jamie and Fred Harwell happy—and for my own peace of mind—I kept trying to get an appointment. This is where another one of those God-instances came into play.

I finally answered Fred's post with a comment to the effect, "I am trying Fred, I am trying!"

The next day, another Facebook friend, Mike Young, who I knew primarily through his relationship with my in-laws—he was a student of and played sports for my father-in-law, Benny "back in the day"—sent me an email. He had close connections with a person on the M.D. Anderson Board of Directors who happened to have connections with Athens and the University of Georgia and he said he could make a call, which he did. Now let me say here and now that if someone else had to wait a little longer to be treated because Mike knew somebody who knew somebody, I am truly sorry. I don't know anything about what strings may or may not have been pulled. All I know is that the next Monday I got a call and will be grateful for that call for the rest of my life.

I had been hoping for an appointment during spring break because I didn't want to miss any more school. I know. Crazy, isn't it? I was fighting to find a cure and stay alive and should not have been worried about missing school—but I was. I wanted Lisa to go with me, too. Let me rephrase that. I needed Lisa to go with me—and she was already off that week. Plus all the literature I read said that patients should be prepared to stay from five to thirty days on their first visit. So I wasn't just hoping for an appointment that week, I was hoping for an appointment at the beginning of that week.

When that first call came, I answered a myriad of questions and the person said she would call me back soon. She did, and told me that I could see a doctor and begin my tests on the Thursday of our spring break. It took a lot of nerve, but I asked her if she could try for the first part of the week. She called me back within the hour and told me that I would begin my testing on Monday, April 2, and see Dr. Lance Pagliara the following morning for my first consultation.

I don't know why my prayers and those lifted up on my behalf are answered and those of other people who are more deserving are not. I just know that I was thankful that these prayers had been answered and I found myself more at peace than I had been in a long time with my situation. All I wanted was to have a chance at the best care possible and I believed that I was about to get that care.

After six months and three subsequent visits, I have seen or experienced nothing to make me change my mind.

But I am getting ahead of the story. No writer worth his weight in printer's ink gives away the ending with so much of the story left to be told. We were talking about the pre-MDA days. I was excited to be going but apprehensive at the same time. Wonderful people who I had never met went to great lengths to try and prepare me for the journey. Total strangers—who were readers or simply friends of friends—sent me long epistles telling me all I needed to know for a short two-day stop or a long six-week stay.

They explained to me how the shuttle worked and told me I should stay at the Rotary House, right there on the campus, if my stay

175

would be a couple of days, but that I should get on a waiting list for a cheaper apartment if I were staying longer. They shared with me the protocols about how to act in the facility and warned me about the emotional attachment I might develop with other people. I never imagined that going to a place for a second opinion could be so complicated. I didn't know how M.D. Anderson Cancer Center operated, either, but I would learn.

Thanks to Mike Young, I had gotten my foot in the door and I was anxious to find out what all the fuss was about. Of course, as it is with every serious medical malady, there was waiting to be done. Time passed slowly between the time we scheduled our first set of tests and the day we finally headed west.

I used that time for reflection, meditation and prayer. You should try it sometime. It doesn't cost anything and I was really able to get in touch with my inner soul. There is a great Jimmy Buffett song—are there any non-great Jimmy Buffett songs?—that contains the line, "I took off for a weekend last month, just to try and recall the whole year; all of the faces and all of the places, wondering where they all disappeared."

I did a lot of pondering during that time—and a lot of time counting my blessings. Being raised in Porterdale was always at the top of that list. I often wonder why, in God's infinite wisdom, He allows some of His children to be born in what seem like God-forsaken places, like the children my daughter, Jenna, travels all over the globe to minister to. Others are born into the lap of luxury with the proverbial silver spoons in their mouths. These folks never want for anything. I was born into the best environment of all. We didn't have much in the way of material things, but we got by and we had everything we needed and were exposed to just enough worldly "stuff" that we grew up knowing what it is to want something and we figured out that the way to have it is to work hard every day.

That knowledge is a lot more valuable than a silver spoon.

Besides, every family in Porterdale had just about what every other family had. We may have been poor, but we never realized it. I am reminded again of my Sociology 101 college professor at the University of Georgia, hallowed be thy name, who introduced me to my classmates as being "raised in poverty, in a north Georgia mill village."

That guy was obviously educated beyond his intelligence. Like I've said before, we weren't poor in Porterdale, we just didn't have any money. There's a great big difference in the two. What we had was the run of that village. We could run out the door at first light and didn't have to be home until the street light came on—or until our mama's called us home to supper. You'd better come flying then or you might get sent to cut a switch.

It might be time for another confession right here. When I was little, my house was sort of a gathering place for my buddies and me. My mama loved having all of us around and it was nothing during the summer time for her to find five or six—or more—little lintheads sleeping all over the beds and couches and even on the screened-in front porch.

When I went to high school, for the first time I made friends with kids who had a lot more "stuff" than my friends in Porterdale or I ever had. They would invite me to spend the night with them and I was amazed at the houses they lived in.

They had carpets and rugs on the floor and light switches on the wall. Our floors had linoleum, if they had any covering at all, and a single light bulb hanging from the center of the room provided what light we had. My friends' houses had closets. We had one chifferobe and one cedar chest to hold my entire family's wardrobes.

And they had walk-in showers. We moved into a house with a claw hammer tub when I was in fifth grade. Before that, we had a bathroom that had been built onto our back porch. Before that, it was a bath with a path. I have taken many a Saturday night bath in a galvanized tub, in water Mama heated on the stove. I hated that, too, because my sister, Myron, always got to go first and she would always—every stinking time—stay in until the water turned cold.

During that time before we headed to Houston, I pondered my youth a lot and my teenage years. My life was pretty much a kaleidoscope during high school. I had many passions. I was a Boy Scout and totally committed to Troop 226. Aubrey Barnes was our Scoutmaster—everybody called him Booney—and I have never known anyone to devote so much time to a group of kids. I tried to live up to my Scout Oath and to the Scout Laws. It is kind of like living up to God's expectations. Sometimes I fell short—but I loved Scouting and would earn my Eagle Award and go on to serve as a Cubmaster and then as Scoutmaster of a troop in Porterdale and even work on Camp Staff at Bert Adams Scout Reservation.

I was Jamison waterfront director for most of those years and have never been happier in my life than the seven summers that I was King of the Jamison Waterfront.

The biggest benefit of working at Bert Adams was the opportunity to meet and work for and love Jack Ross Bowden Jr. Jack was so much fun to be around and he taught me so much about living life to the utmost. Jack knew more about boys and young men that anyone I had ever known, before or since. There was no squabble he couldn't mediate with soft words, accompanied by a freshly pulled watermelon split open with a Buck knife and passed around the room.

We lost Uncle Jack way too soon and I thought about him a lot during that late spring and wondered if he would be proud of who I had become.

My other passion during high school was basketball. I loved the game and played Junior Varsity in the ninth grade. That's when our coach, the legendary Ronald Bradley, who has won more games than anyone who ever coached in Georgia, realized that I would make All America—as a manager. He was right, and I did. It is pointless to try and explain how much Ronald and Jan Bradley have meant to me during my entire life. It would take an entire book—and maybe I'll write that book one day. "We're from Newton; Couldn't be Prouder."

Catchy title, huh? But I pondered the good times I had with the Bradleys and with my teammates and counted as a blessing the fact that I was able to count them all as friends—even Brenda, I hope, who is a little mad at me because of something I posted online about the Auburn Creed the night scholar-athletes Cam Newton and Nick Fairley dismantled my beloved Georgia football team. Maybe she'll forgive me.

In fact, I have a lot of people I need to ask forgiveness from and I pondered these people in my heart. I thought about Blake's comment and did not want to be weighed in the balance and found wanting. I prayed. I read scriptures. I examined my life and steeled myself for the future, determined that I would begin immediately that Christian walk that John Wesley described as "a journey toward perfection."

I pondered my relationship with my wife and was sorry about so many things—so many times we hadn't communicated, so many times I had failed to show how much I appreciated her, so many regrets—we all have them, don't we? I promised myself that I would cherish each and every day God allows us to be together.

I pondered our children. I may not have the three greatest kids on earth, but I have never found three that I would swap them for. I realized, during my pondering, that the Lord God Almighty, in His infinite wisdom, put Lisa and me together because only by our union could the three magnificent human beings who would become Jamie, Jackson and Jenna Huckaby been procreated.

Jamie is a typical first child. We don't call her the princess for nothing. She is extremely intelligent and earned a Doctor of Pharmacy degree when she was 23. I am certain that I raised Jamie right. She is about to be married. Her wedding is scheduled to take place in the UGA Chapel and the reception will be on Herty Field—Georgia's first gridiron. The rehearsal dinner will be in the President's Skybox at Sanford Stadium. I told you I raised her right!

My daddy started taking me to Georgia games when I was knee-high to a grasshopper. We couldn't afford tickets. We would sit on the railroad tracks and peer down onto the field of play. Our tailgate was mayonnaise sandwiches wrapped in waxed paper. Once in a great while Mama would send us with a shoebox full of fried chicken and a few deviled eggs. I would drink sweet iced tea from a Mason jar. I guess Daddy drank water because the contents of his Mason jar were always clear. I thought every time we went, "Man, if only I could get inside that stadium one time."

I have been inside that stadium now, thank you—and when Jamie was a little girl, she would be my date for the games. Lisa worked weekends and stayed home with Jamie during the week. I spent the weekends with her, and when the Dawgs played between the hedges, I would dress her in red and black and we would go to the games.

I taught her all about Georgia football long before she should have been able to comprehend.

Her passion for the game backfired on me one time, however. It was the Fourth of July weekend and Dan Brokaw was leading one of his magnificent concerts at the eleven o'clock church service. This one was filled with patriotic music. The choir was singing the Battle Hymn of the Republic and Brother Dan had built a huge crescendo as the choir held a long note after "Glory! Glory! Halleluiah . . ."

And Jamie Leigh, who was two and a half, at the time, stood up on her pew and shouted, "And to hell with Georgia Tech!"

Church was over. They finally let me rejoin this past August. I'm not sure if I can bring Jamie with me or not.

I pondered Jamie's life and found myself wondering if I could have been a better dad for her and I found myself wondering if I would live to see her get married. I wondered if I would know my grandkids or if they would know anything about their grandfather.

Then there was Jackson, our only son. He might just be the best person I know. He isn't anything like me, and for that I give thanks. He is kind and calm and laid back. He is also intelligent and loving and tenderhearted. If Baden Powell had met Jackson before founding the Boy Scout movement, he would have added some of his qualities to the Scout Law.

Jackson and I had lots of fun when he was a kid. Santa Claus always brought him the best toys. I don't know how St. Nick knew, but Jackson got all the things I wished I could have gotten for Christmas, things that just never quite found their way into the mill village houses—slot car racers and electric trains and huge cases of K'NEX building sets. We built a roller coaster and a Ferris wheel and I don't know what all. Jackson got little cars with motors and rockets—did we ever have fun building those rockets.

When it came time to play sports, I got to coach his teams in basketball and soccer. He was a gym rat and rarely, if ever, missed a basketball practice or game when I was coaching the girls' teams at Edwards Middle School and Heritage High.

Jackson was raised a Bulldog, too, of course, and I was thrilled when he was accepted to UGA. Jackson made 1400 on his SAT and

I wasn't sure that would be enough for him to get into Georgia. Two of us used to get in for that. In fact, when I got my acceptance letter in 1970, it was addressed to Darrell Huckaby or Current Occupant. It ain't that way anymore.

UGA agreed with Jackson and now he is one of the newest math teachers in our fair state. I am actually shocked that one of my children majored in math. He certainly didn't get his aptitude for figures from me. Come to think of it, his mother's not that bright, either. I took exactly one math class during my undergraduate days. It was college algebra from Colonel Stanley—I think he must have earned his rank under General Lee in the Army of Northern Virginia. I wasn't a real good math student, but Colonel Stanley agreed to give me a D if I agreed never to take one of his classes again. It was a win-win for both of us.

Jackson didn't enroll in college with the intention of being a math teacher. He started out in landscape architecture. One spring evening, I got a late-night call from my cousin Carolyn, whose son, Howell, had earned an LAR degree from UGA. We lost Howell in a tragic automobile crash and my cousin endows a scholarship in his honor. She had been to the annual banquet to do just that the evening she called me.

I was surprised to learn that my son's name had been on the agenda that night. He was to have received an award as the top sophomore student in his program and, according to Carolyn, was not there to receive it. I immediately called him to ask him why.

He stammered around a bit and finally told me that he had changed majors and didn't feel right accepting the award when he wasn't going to stay in the program. "Why didn't you tell me you were changing majors?" was my next question.

"I didn't want you to yell at me," was his response.

"Don't be silly," I said. "Why would I do that? What did you change to?"

He told me education. I yelled at him.

And then I asked him why he wanted to be a teacher. His explanation humbled me.

He said that all they talked about in business classes was "making money" and he said that making money didn't interest him that much. That's an easy position to hold when your parents have always given you all the money you've needed.

He went on to say that he started trying to figure out what would make him happy and make him feel like he was making a difference in the world. He started listing the people he knew that seemed happy—and the people who had positively impacted his life.

They were all teachers.

He specifically mentioned his band director, Greg Gajownik, and his statistics teacher, Maggie Tramantano, and one of his social studies teachers, Jim Hauck. Then he said, "Everywhere we go people come up to you and say you taught them at this school or that school and they all seem to think so much of you and they all tell you what a difference you made in their lives. I want to make a difference in people's lives, too."

What could I say to counter that?

You are right. Nothing.

As I pondered in my heart Jackson's childhood, just as I had with Jamie, I wondered if my parenting had been sufficient and if he understood how much I truly loved him.

Then there was Jenna, or Boo Boo, as we had always called her. I have always said that she might just be the best of the bunch. She is a dynamic, passionate person who loves life. She is a thrill-seeker and burns her candle on both ends. She is wide out, all day and all night. I don't know where she gets that from, but it worries me. She wants to do everything there is to do, and a lot of times I just have to plead with her to slow down and give up on some of her many expectations.

Every time I suggest that she not do something she says, "You did that."

Every time I have to tell her that I have done a lot of things that I don't want her to do.

They say that a rolling stone gathers no moss. We won't ever have to worry about Jenna Huckaby having a mossy back, I can assure you of that. She was in New Mexico, saving the American West, when I had my robotic surgery. She was in the jungles of Benin, in West Africa, during the summer of 2012—sleeping under the stars, living from hand to mouth, sharing the love of Jesus Christ with the poorest of the poor without ever expecting or hoping to get anything in return but a smile.

As I thought about Jenna I wondered if I had given her enough attention when she was a child. She was so much like me and so fiercely independent, but we never sat down and communicated that much. I knew she knew I loved her, but I wondered, as with the others, if she knew how much.

There was a lot of pondering to be done, understand, and a lot of blessings to be counted, a lot of forgiveness to be asked for and a lot of reflection on how I could come to be the person that I had been created to be.

So many people's names crossed my mind during these long sessions of reflection and meditation and prayer. How can one person have been touched by so many other lives?

Take Tony Gray, the sage of Salem Road. Tony and I went to high school together and he is the only teacher at Heritage who has served on the faculty every year the school has been open. He is the last man standing. Tony, simply put, is one of the best people I know. I started at Heritage in 1999, and during the first semester, just before Christmas, my mother died. Tony was one of the first people through the door at the visitation. When I expressed my appreciation at his coming he said, "This is a tough one, here. I wouldn't be anywhere else."

I know for a solid gold fact that I was never far from Tony's mind—or prayers—during this entire ordeal. If I needed someone to talk to, I could approach Tony without fear of anything I told him being repeated or expounded upon. When I didn't feel like talking, Tony completely understood.

Tony likes to ride Harley-Davidsons and when we travel around the country I like to find unusual Harley-Davidson T-shirts to bring back to him. I don't know if they have Harley Tees in heaven but if they do—and I get there before him—I am sending him one, somehow.

183

Lisa Byrd is another teacher friend. Even though her own mother was in the process of dying from cancer during the spring of that awful year, she still found the strength and energy and courage to help keep my spirits up.

Once you start pondering, it is hard to stop. There was the Thomson trio, the great coach, John Barnett, and his buddies, Gene Walker and Ralph Thomson. They would ride over from eastern Georgia frequently and sit on my couch and regale me with stories about some of the wackiest people in the American South.

I met John while taking an AP seminar in Athens one summer. We found a lot of common ground and hit it off immediately. My kids, in fact, refer to John as "that man that is just like you." When he and I get together, you'd better have on high waders and a pair of goggles because the BS is going to fly and it is going to get deep— way deep.

I relived my life that spring and I regretted a lot of the things I had done, and regretted even more alot of the things that I had not done. Through it all, I focused on the inspired Word of God as recorded in the scriptures and as I realized that God's grace was, indeed, sufficient for me, I began to experience that blessed peace that passes all understanding. I knew that, whatever I had done, God was willing to forgive me and had, in fact, sent His only son to die for the atonement of my many sins. If that isn't love, the ocean is dry and there are no stars in the sky. Yeah, I stole that from a song.

I found peace because I knew everything was in God's control and that when I died, I would live eternally with Him. That's a pretty good feeling. If you don't have that peace, let me know. I can help you find it.

Now don't hear something I'm not saying. I still wanted to live—and still do. I have a lot of unfinished business down here.

I'm like the little boy I had in my Sunday school class one time. I asked who all wanted to go to heaven. Every child raised his hand except Kenneth.

"Kenneth," I said. "You don't want to go to heaven when you die?"

His hand shot straight up and he said, "Yes, sir, Mr. Darrell. I want to go to heaven when I die. I thought you were getting up a bunch to go right now!"

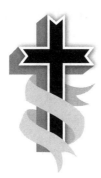

CHAPTER TWENTY SEVEN

You have to be able to laugh if you are going to survive cancer. It's a good thing that I like to laugh and that I have always been able to laugh at myself. When I would find myself in the doldrums—and I did spend a lot of time down there—I would try to look at the lighter side of life. Writing my column was a wonderful outlet.

I became a newspaper columnist quite by happenstance. I mean, I didn't sit down and write a series of columns and submit them to an editor somewhere. I had written a book, Need Two, and I would send columns into the Atlanta Journal-Constitution for publication. It was sort of a freelance gig. I quit doing that, however, when Cynthia Tucker took over the editorial pages of that paper. I couldn't recognize anything I had written when she got through with it.

Then one day I got a call from Alice Queen, wanting to know if I would write a column for our local hometown paper, the Rockdale Citizen. At first I said no, because I had read that the Citizen's new editor had previously worked for the Lexington, Massachusetts, paper. The last thing I needed was to have some hairy-legged Yankee woman busting my chops over what I had written about the American South in my weekly column.

Ms. Queen was persistent, however, and finally convinced me to at least come in and talk to her. By this time, truth be told, I had realized that her accent was much too sweet and soft and Southern to belong to somebody from above the Mason-Dixon Line. When I learned that she was a good old gal from Montezuma, Georgia, I was all in.

Alice Queen changed my life when she asked me to write a weekly column in her newspaper. Pretty soon, I was writing twice a week and then three times and then in other papers. Maybe one day I will retire from education and write full time and a lot of people will know about my work. For now, I am happy to be a small fish in a small pond and Alice has become a true friend. She pretends she doesn't even notice when I feel so bad from my disease and the treatments that I doctor up a column from 1998 or 2003 and submit it for publication.

Many readers call me out, but Alice pretends not to notice.

On days when I feel the worst, I can sit down at the keyboard and hammer out something that makes me laugh or remember happier days and I feel better. When I get responses from readers saying that what I wrote struck a chord with them, I feel better still.

I am not sure if Reader's Digest was right. I am not positively certain that laughter is the very best medicine, but it is certainly good for what ails you.

The Moby in the Morning Show gave me another outlet and a world of support. My whole family used to listen to Moby when he was on Kicks 101.5 FM, back in the 1990s. Then they fired my boy for sounding "too country." How can you sound "too country" for a country music station? Anyway, I heard through the grapevine that Moby was back on the air with a syndicated show.

I couldn't pick it up in my house but I went to his website and, lo and behold, right there on the front page of his website was a piece entitled, "30 Things All Georgians Should Know." It had some right good advice in that article, too. Things like, Stone Mountain is the biggest carving in the world and that the guy who carved Mount Rushmore started carving the one on Stone Mountain but gave up because the granite was too hard.

Other things were in the article like, "Crack cocaine has done more damage to Atlanta than Sherman ever thought of" and that "If it weren't for a Georgian, Crawford W. Long of Jefferson, open heart surgery would hurt like hell."

That sort of stuff. You may have seen it. It has circulated around the internet for years. I was very familiar with it because I wrote it—in 1995. It was published in my third book, Grits is Groceries. But was I ever given credit as the author? Noooo.

And there Mr. Moby was, featuring my work on his website. It just so happened that I ran into Moby in Athens and told them that I had a bone to pick with him. I explained the situation and he apologized. He then asked me to call him the next Wednesday and read my column on his radio show. And I have been calling Moby every Wednesday since and sharing my foolishness and my outrage with all our radio cousins.

I love doing my "What the Huck" segment on his show and have made some great connections. Moby has become like a brother to me. During my entire journey, he has been supportive and has petitioned his listeners for prayers on my behalf. Moby is just one more of those folks I couldn't have gotten through this without.

Martha Mann is another, speaking of laughter being good for your soul. Martha and Bobby Mann are members of my tailgate group and best friends with my in-laws and some kind of branch kin on Lisa's side of the family. Martha, I believe, is close to eighty years old, but is going on about seventeen. She is the youngest older person I know and keeps me hopping all the time. Her husband, Bob, was a paratrooper in the Army and claims to have made fourteen take-offs in an airplane before he ever experienced a landing. The other thirteen times he says he jumped out. Bob also worked on the Alaskan pipeline for a couple of years and has tons of stories about his adventures. Whenever I needed a pick-me-up, Martha and Bob were happy to oblige.

When things got really bleak, I would walk down the long hallway of our school to Caroline Ingle's room and we would commiserate about how much it sucked having cancer. Caroline's then-fiancé and now-husband, Robert St. John, would often wander in and join the conversation. Robert's philosophy was "if you're going to have cancer, you might as well make the most of it," and was constantly encouraging me to seek out better parking places and restaurant tables and seats at ballgames. "Just tell them you have cancer," he always said. "They'll let you sit anywhere!"

One of the things Caroline and I liked to talk about were all the miracle cures out there. Now please understand this. I am not trying to be ugly and I appreciate every single person who offered me any advice whatsoever about dealing with my illness. I know that some of the suggested diets and health plans that folks have submitted to me have genuine merit. I am just not self-disciplined enough to follow up on them—no, not even if it saves my life.

My former girlfriend, Tammy Harrison, for instance, went to great deal of time and effort to write out a list of protocols that would help me stay healthier longer, even if it did not cure my cancer. When I say she went to a lot of trouble, I mean it. And I appreciated it. I know she had no agenda other than to help me recover and everything she said made perfect sense, medically and scientifically. I just couldn't bring myself to stay on her protocols. That doesn't mean I didn't appreciate her efforts. I did—and do.

Other folks were not so in tune with science and nutrition, however. There is a recent widower in our community that to this day insists, every time he sees me, that there is a cure for cancer that the doctors are keeping secret because they are making too much money treating cancer patients.

Another person insisted that all I had to do to cure my cancer was eat half-a-lemon every day. That's it. No more cancer. Guaranteed. I am afraid that one won't fly. Few days have passed since I grew teeth that I haven't had at least half-a-lemon and I got cancer anyway.

But I appreciated the sentiment and the time it took for the person to contact me. Just about everyone I met knew a sure-fire way for me to cure my cancer, even though they didn't know exactly what type of cancer I had or where it had metastasized or the severity or anything else about my specific case. They just knew that they had read on the internet that drinking kale and carrot juice cocktails every day for eleven months would destroy cancer or that cancer could not live in an alkaline environment or that their next-door neighbor's friend's boyfriend's cousin's grandma only had an hour-and-a-half to live and they started using this-that-or-the-other and was completely cured and now they are an eighty-nine-year-old Olympian.

I know. I know. I am making light. I don't mean to be and I do know there are many substantiated cases of people using alternative methods of fighting their cancer and being cured. Jamie's fiancé's father is a perfect example. After evaluating all the suggestions, however, I simply decided that a medical solution would be the best path for me to follow—that and prayer. I didn't resent people trying to get me to try other things. I knew they had my best interests at heart and I appreciated the fact that they cared.

I even had people follow me out of the post office or chase me down leaving the bank just so they could share their miracle cure. One woman had been stalking me for weeks and had a notebook full of information. She almost ran over me in the Publix parking lot. She almost killed me so she could save my life.

The only people who upset me were the ones who tried to sell me their snake oil. Buy Juice-Plus from me and you will be well in a week, that sort of thing.

One woman, who will remain nameless, saw me every day for a year and a half and never as much as asked how I was feeling. Then she became part of a pyramid-type sales force to sell some sort of vitamin water and she was suddenly oh, so concerned. She really wanted to bring me the information because she had a friend who had Stage 4 terminal cancer and started drinking the water and was completely cured in a week. "In fact," she said, "I have three friends that happened to."

Right. And I am a midget Russian astronaut.

As Mark Twain said, "Man is the only animal that blushes—or needs to."

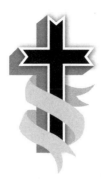

Chapter Twenty Eight

One of the best things about teaching for a living is spring break. Practically every spring since we have been married, Lisa and I have joined a large group of her family and friends and gone camping at Jekyll Island, on the Georgia coast. It is always an idyllic week devoted to bike riding, good food and long nights around the campfire.

This year, however, we would have a completely different type of spring break. Lisa and I would be forgoing the beach and heading to Houston, hoping against hope that we would find some great answers to the questions that had been bothering us so. Honesty compels me to admit that while I had been growing closer and closer in my relationship with God for months and while my faith had given me a more positive outlook and had allowed me to become much more confident about my outcome, I was a hot mess in the days leading up to our trip to M.D. Anderson.

I just didn't like the idea of not knowing how long I would be asked to stay. Lisa and I were driving, and we had made reservations for three days in Houston—but what if I had to stay longer? Would Lisa just drive the car home and leave me there alone? Would she have to fly home and leave me there with the car? Maybe they would let me drive her home and then fly back. Where would I stay if they kept me for a long series of treatments? How in the world would we afford to pay for the trip and an extended stay if it came to that?

Oh, I had worked myself up into a state by the time we were ready to go, let me tell you. Remember the verse in the Bible where we are told to worry about nothing but to pray in all situations? I remembered it; I just couldn't bring myself to follow it.

Consider the lilies of the field. Remember the sparrows. I knew all that. I had a tough time living it that week.

Lisa and I were to leave on Saturday morning. We would drive about halfway, find a place to stop for the night and then drive on into Houston on Sunday. My first appointment was scheduled for Monday morning. On that Friday afternoon, Cherie Fambrough and Holle Stapp came by the house to drop off a basketful of goodies. When I say a basketful, I mean a basket full.

They had packed all the things I like. Those little Coca-Colas in the green bottles that taste so good when they are iced down and a little crust forms on the top, peanuts, cashews, crackers, and Holle's special gorp, which is a mixture of sweet and salty with M&Ms thrown in for good measure. They also included neck pillows and blankets and gift cards and everything you can imagine and a few things you never could.

I suppose I should reveal here that Cherie is another one of my favorite people on earth. I taught her two beautiful and intelligent daughters, Jada and Kara, and Cherie has been a huge supporter of mine ever since. Holle and her husband, Clay, along with their kids, Jeremy, Matt, and Morgan, are our travel buddies and like an extension of our own family. It was an emotional thing to have these wonderful folks drop by to see me—and the gifts they brought were so incredibly thoughtful.

I welcomed them into the kitchen, but when Holle asked me a question, I just lost total control of myself. It was the worst twenty minutes of the entire ordeal to that point. I couldn't talk, I couldn't speak, I couldn't control my emotions or my tears, and I had no idea why I couldn't.

Holle, who on many trips has experienced the wrath of certain parties for not staying on schedule, said that it was because I am so used to being in charge and now I was in a situation in which I had no control at all. It was quite a profound statement, and she was absolutely right. After they left, while I was still dealing with the embarrassment of my outburst, I sat myself down and had a little talk. "Self," I said, "Holle is right. You are not in control, but you know who is. God is in control and you have got to quit worrying and put your faith in Him. He has never let you down before and He is not going to start now. You have been going all over Georgia preaching faith and assurance and telling people that all is well with your soul. Now you have to live it."

That was good little talk, and after another hour or so of uncontrollable sobbing, I got myself together and did exactly what I told myself to do. When morning came, I felt more composed than I had in months. Lisa and I put our bags in the trunk of the car and Cherie and Holle's basket in the back seat and we hit the road.

I love to travel. I always dreamed of retiring from teaching and getting a job as a travel writer. We have taken our children to all fifty states—camping on most of our trips. You haven't lived until you have pulled a pop-up camper behind a Dodge Caravan to California and back, accompanied by a menopausal wife and three teenagers.

I've done it twice—so far.

When we travel, we have a special CD we listen to. As we pulled out of our driveway that morning, I slid it into our player and we were greeted by Kay Starr singing Side by Side. We have begun every trip for the last thirty years with Kay Starr singing Side by Side, but the words never struck me like they did this time.

"Oh we ain't got a barrel of money, maybe we're ragged and funny, but we'll travel along, singing our song, side by side. Don't know what's coming tomorrow, maybe its trouble and sorrow, but we'll travel the road, sharing our load—side by side."

Suddenly, I felt like singing—so I did.

It's a long way from Atlanta to Houston, but the thing is, New Orleans is right on the way—or at least it can be. Except it couldn't be for us this time because the Kentucky Wildcats were playing the Louisville Cardinals in the semi-finals of the NCAA championship tournament. Consequently, the Bluegrass State had taken over the Crescent City. We were lucky to find a room up on Interstate 10, but we made do.

We made the most of the next day's drive. We stopped and toured the LSU campus and said hello to Mike the Tiger. He lives in his own private zoo, right next to the football stadium. Thinking of Robert St. John's advice to always play the cancer card, I sweet-talked a lady who was manning the gate to the stadium while waiting for the LSU coaches to come in and grade film from the previous day's spring game to give Lisa and me our own private tour of Death Valley. It didn't look so intimidating at ten o'clock on a Sunday morning.

While we were in Baton Rouge, we visited the state capitol and saw where the Kingfish, Huey Long, was gunned down in cold blood and we took off our shoes and walked in the Mississippi River. It was such a pleasant day that we almost forgot where we were going and why.

Almost—but not quite.

I know I keep going on and on about random people who did so much to make this journey a little more manageable, but like Larry Munson said after the Buck Belue-to-Lindsay Scott miracle play in the famous Gator Bowl, "I didn't mean to beg Lindsay to run, but I had to," I don't mean to just keep mentioning so many people and so many kindnesses, but I have to. I am amazed at how many of them there are, and for every person or act or deed that I am mentioning, I am leaving out a dozen or two dozen more. I am trying, in my own inadequate way, to illustrate how far the love of God can spread. It has taken every kindness, every card and letter, every Facebook "like" and, most importantly, every prayer for me to get where I have gotten.

The acts of kindness were just beginning when we got to M.D. Anderson.

I drove the entire way and honesty compels me to admit that I was worn out when we finally pulled into Houston. I was not too tired to argue with my navigator about her driving instructions, but I was pretty wasted when we finally arrived at the Rotary House, where we were staying.

I felt at home at M.D. Anderson from the time we pulled into the driveway of the adjacent hotel. The valet was not at all pushy and waited patiently while we made sure we had everything we needed out of the car. As soon as we entered the lobby, a hostess greeted us and took us immediately to the welcome center. She sat us down and went over my medical records and all of my impending appointments. She explained how to find our way around the enormous compound of buildings and gave us a short rundown on restaurants and shopping facilities in the area. The whole process was amazingly smooth.

Next we checked into our room. No problem there, either. The lady who checked us in didn't even ask for a credit card—just my ID and patient number. Yes, they wanted my patient number at the hotel desk. Every person who stays at the M.D. Anderson Rotary House must be a patient or a caregiver accompanying a patient. We went up to our room, on the eleventh floor. We had a great view with a giant king-sized bed and a large flat-screen high-definition television. The only thing that made the Rotary House different from any luxury hotel I had ever stayed in were the bars on the shower and toilet—that and the relatively low price, of course.

I collapsed on the bed and took a nap before getting ready for our dinner date. Now hang with me here while I tell you about Texas A&M Aggies. They are not cut from the same bolt of cloth as most people.

I got hooked up with Texas A&M about five years ago when I had an encounter on Jekyll Island with a young man who had just come home from his second tour of duty in Iraq. He and his family were enjoying a little weekend getaway. I was appreciative of his service and his family's sacrifice and wrote about it. It went viral among Aggies everywhere and I got hundreds of responses from people wanting to tell me more good things about their school and its traditions. I then wrote about that and got thousands more responses. Eventually I was invited out to College Station, Texas, and they really rolled out the welcome mat for me.

Two of the Aggies who were instrumental in arranging my trip to the campus, Kyle and Dee Ann Jones, learned that I was coming to Houston for treatments. They drove the 120 miles from their home to Houston to greet Lisa and me and take us out to supper that night. That's the kind of folks Aggies are.

I continued to be amazed by MDA the entire time I was there. Nothing against any of the other places I sought treatment, but I was able to get done in two days out there what it took several weeks to get done back home. We met with Dr. Lance Pagliaro first thing Monday morning. As soon as I learned that he would be my doctor, I looked him up—on the Internet, of course—and learned that he had been one of the go-to guys for years for advanced prostate cancer.

What it didn't say in his online biography was that Dr. Pagliaro is confined to a wheelchair. Lisa and I were surprised when he knocked on our examining room door and wheeled himself in. I was immediately impressed with his demeanor and his no-nonsense, get-right-to-the-point manner. He interviewed me thoroughly about my case, which meant that he asked me more questions than I could answer. Luckily, Lisa was with me and knew everything I didn't—which has been the case for three decades now.

Dr. Pagliaro was non-committal about whether he would take my case or not. He sent us to the lab for a blood test and told us to enjoy Houston and come back the next day. He had scheduled bone scans for me along with a few other tests, but since we had just had them done a couple of weeks earlier at Rockdale Medical Center in Conyers, we got to leave film of those results with him and didn't have to repeat them. Thank the Lord and RMC's CEO, Deborah Armstrong, for large favors.

I wanted to go for a swim and lay around in the hot tub all afternoon—yes, the Rotary House has a pool and a hot tub. Lisa wanted to take a walk and examine all the hospitals in the Texas Medical Center area. We went for a walk.

Y'all! You wouldn't believe the bright, modern gleaming hospitals that are concentrated in that area of Houston: Texas Women's Hospital, Texas Children's Hospital, Methodist Hospital, Baylor Medical, Shriner's Hospital, St. Luke's—I could go on and on and on. Of course, Lisa wanted to see inside all of them, so we did.

That night, another old friend, Kyle Carpenter, came over to take us out to dinner. Kyle is the ex-boyfriend of our daughter, Jamie, but we still love him and his family. He is in medical school at Baylor University and were we ever glad to see him. He took us to one of the best Mexican restaurants ever. I had the fajitas. Lisa had the margaritas. It was a good night.

Honesty compels me to admit that I didn't sleep well that night, and it had nothing to do with the fact that I had watched Kentucky win the NCAA Championship on television. Visions of all of the patients I'd seen all day were dancing in my head when I turned in.

You've heard the old adage, I was sad because I didn't have any shoes; then I met a man who had no feet. If that isn't an old adage, it should be. That's the way I felt as I wandered the halls of M.D. Anderson and enjoyed the hospitality of the Rotary House that first day. Imagine an eleven-story downtown hotel where every single person staying there has cancer. Most were much further along than me. There were so many people who were obviously fighting for their lives—people who had lost their hair from chemotherapy, people who had to have personal oxygen tanks to breathe, people who were in wheelchairs and had lost limbs—people who were barely holding on to their last shred of hope.

Try as I might I could not help but wonder how long it would be until I was in their shoes—or their wheelchairs—or if Dr. Pagliaro had hope of a cure and a complete recovery waiting for me the next day. I finally drifted off into a fitful sleep.

The next morning, we were anxious to get over to the Mays Clinic and hear the results of the all-telling PSA test. Every result we had gotten from a PSA test had resulted in disappointment. The PSA was always rising and it was always rising more quickly than we expected. The news this time was the same.

The day before, Dr. Pagliaro had questioned us about why we had driven all the way to Houston seeking treatment. He suggested that we might want to hear his opinion and then seek treatment back in Atlanta, for the sake of convenience. He didn't bring that option up at our second meeting.

He informed us that the PSA was indeed still rising. It had doubled within the past month. He then laid out our best options for treatment. There were two. We could begin hormone therapy immediately or we could begin hormone therapy in conjunction with a clinical drug trial that was just getting underway.

The hormone treatment was the same suggested by the doctor at Emory whose bedside manner left much to be desired. It would con- sist of regular injections of a drug called Lupron, which destroys all the testosterone in your body, since prostate cancer feeds off testosterone. Another name for the Lupron treatments is chemical castration. If that is hard to read, imagine how hard it is to consent to.

Dr. P was very blunt about Lupron's effects. He said that my sex drive and my ability to have intercourse would diminish within a couple of weeks. He said that the drug would cause my bones to deteriorate, give me frequent hot flashes, just like a woman going through meno- pause, and would cause fatigue and lethargy. He said it would cause my upper body musculature to decline, to be replaced by fat tissue. He also said that, since my cancer had already metastasized, I would be on the drug permanently unless a new treatment or cure was discovered. He said that the initial injection would definitely lower my PSA and men- tioned 2.4 as a potential target score after 12 weeks. He said that he had many patients who had been on Lupron for ten years or more.

I asked him if it were likely that a person with my type of cancer— the microscopic kind that had survived surgery and radiation after early detection—was likely to remain diminished on Lupron for ten years. He looked me in the eye and said flatly, "No." I had read the research.

I knew that it might work for twelve to eighteen months, or that it might not work at all.

As I said, he did offer us an opportunity to be a part of a clinical trial for a proposed drug that stimulates the body to actually fight off and kill the cancer cells—but that drug was also permanent. Once you introduced it into the body, you couldn't back off or your immune system would be compromised. The potential side effects seemed much worse than anything I had experienced with my cancer. The doctor left us alone for a while to discuss the options. We decided to pass on that particular trial and wait for a more promising one.

When Dr. Pagliaro came back in we told him our decision and he told us that the nurse would be in shortly to administer the first injection. Again, M.D. Anderson is amazing. The doctor in Atlanta had told us that we needed to get the Lupron pre-certified by our insurance company and order the shot a couple of weeks in advance.

True to Dr. P's word, the nurse came in sooner rather than later, with a great big needle that I was certain was going to smart. You might think that getting an injection is not a big deal, but I have never liked needles and getting an injection that is going to permanently take away the physical part of your manhood is not an easy thing—at least it wasn't for me.

Lisa, on the other hand, had been waiting for this day for years. She took out her iPhone and videoed the whole process. It will probably wind up in the Smithsonian someday—or at the very least on YouTube with the one of Prince Harry frolicking in the nude. If you ask nicely she would probably give you a peak for free.

I tried to be a trooper though. I dropped trou and leaned over the examination table and told her to have at it. She told me it would hurt. It did. But it was over quickly. Afterward, the doctor came back in, shook my hand, and told me that we were free to go and that he would see me in twelve weeks.

I felt a bit melancholy as we headed back to our room, which was reserved for the rest of the week. Since it was not yet noon and since our business there was done, for the time being, we packed our bags, checked out of the hotel, had the valet bring our car around—and headed for New Orleans.

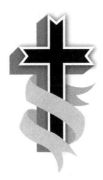

CHAPTER TWENTY NINE

I had peace in my heart as we left Houston and headed east that I had not enjoyed for a long time. I had already made peace with God and was ready for whatever He had planned for me. I knew from the beginning of this ordeal that my name was long ago written in the Book of Life—along with a birth date and an expiration date. I wanted to hang around down here a while longer, but if it was not to be, then it was not to be. So, for a while things had been well with my soul.

But now I was at peace mentally, too, because I knew that I had done everything within my power and had left no stone unturned—except an all-kale diet that I really didn't think I could do anyway. My spirits began to pick up and the further we drove, the more I looked forward to one more visit to the City that Care Forgot with the love of my life. Honesty compels me to admit that I believed this would be my last visit to New Orleans, just as I believed the previous Christmas would be my last Christmas and that my fifty-ninth birthday would be my last birthday.

God proved me wrong on the birthday and Christmas counts and now I am hopeful that I'll spend a lot more time on Bourbon Street. But on this particular day, I was certain it would be my last trip so I was determined to hit all our favorite spots. We did, too.

We didn't have any magic coupons this time, but we did find a special rate at the Iberville Suites, which shares an entrance, a lounge, and a pool with the Ritz-Carlton right next door. We were rubbing shoulders in the hot tub with the glitz set and they were paying four times the amount we were. I also learned when I looked at my Rotary House receipt a little more closely that the reason they hadn't asked for a credit card when I checked in was because our ex-cousin-in-law, Phil Bartholomew, had called ahead and picked up our tab.

Hebrews 13:2 warns us, "Do not neglect to show hospitality to strangers, for by doing that some have entertained angels without knowing it." I have learned many times during this perilous journey through the valley of the shadow of death that the previous message cuts both ways. I have been entertained by angels time and time again without even knowing it. I am certain many readers of this tome will grow weary of reading about countless random people who have shown me kindness during this ordeal, but I continue to mention them because everyone I have mentioned—and the countless folks I have failed to mention—are doing the work of God right here on earth. They serve as a reminder to me—and hopefully you—of how we are instructed to live our lives.

As Iris Standard read on that memorable Easter Sunday, "Lord, you know I love you."

"Take care of my lambs."

I am a lamb of God and the Lord is my shepherd. He has some wonderful helpers down here on earth.

Back to New Orleans. We strolled down Bourbon Street, almost enjoying the stench that not even Hurricane Katrina could wash away. We went in and out of the art galleries on Royal Street, rode the St. Charles Streetcar, ate raw oysters at Felix's—at least I did—and enjoyed a Ferdi special and bread pudding at Mother's Restaurant. That evening we dined at Commander's Palace. Frommer's once called Commander's the best restaurant in the world, which is saying something because there are lots of restaurants in the world. I have eaten there several times and have never found a reason to disagree with Frommer's.

After dinner, Lisa had a Flaming Hurricane at Pat O'Brien's and, of course, we topped off the evening with beignets and café au lait at Café du Monde in the French Market. To top off a perfect day in the Crescent City, we fell asleep in one another's arms while a magnificent thunderstorm pounded the old-fashioned windows of our hotel suite.

Life was good that day.

When we arrived home, I was determined to live every remaining day of my life. I still taught school every day. I felt pretty fresh each morning but was worn out by the end of the day. I would go home after school and take a nap, and then I would get up and walk a couple of miles, cook supper if Lisa was at work, and spend the evening writing, reading, and reflecting.

I spent a lot of time in God's word. I had once read how Billy Graham described his Bible reading regimen. He said that he reads five Psalms each day and then one chapter from the book of Proverbs, followed by several chapters from the Old Testament and several from the New Testament. When he gets to the end he starts over. If it is good enough for Billy Graham, it is good enough for this old Porterdale linthead. I started following the same regimen—most nights.

I found a lot of comfort in the book of Psalms. King David might have been an adulterer and a murderer and a liar, but he was a man after God's own heart. I thought if God could use David with all his faults, I knew God could use me, too.

I turned in most nights at 9:30. I didn't go immediately to sleep, however. That was my quiet time and in the privacy of my own bedroom, I spent a lot of time with God. Much of it was spent counting my many blessings. Strangely enough, I counted contracting cancer as a blessing because having the disease truly did bring me closer to God. It caused me to examine and reorder my life, and my life needed reexamining and reordering. Having cancer brought Lisa and me closer together because we had to talk about things we had never really talked about before and we had to take care of one another. And having cancer made me more pliable to God's will. I had always avoided turning my life completely over to God because, as Holle Stapp had noted the day before we left for Houston, I like to be in control. I don't like anyone telling me what to do.

During the weeks and months following our first visit to M.D. Anderson, I put my life completely in the hands of my Savior. I surrendered all to Him and I asked Him every night for guidance. I pleaded with God for discernment in my life. I made sure God knew that I wanted to use whatever time I had left on earth to glorify Him and wanted to make sure that I fulfilled my purpose, whatever it might be, for being on this earth to begin with.

As always, God continued to be good to me. I could feel His forgiveness enveloping me and the power of the Holy Spirit engulfing me and I knew, for possibly the first time since I heard Dr. Entrekin tell me that he was pretty sure I had cancer, that everything was going to be OK.

I asked for direction and God continued to provide that direction. The entire spring was filled with one God-incidence after another. Seemingly random occurrences seemed to bring many loose ends in my life together. It really was as if I could see through a dark glass. I didn't know my precise destination, but I knew that I was being guided in the right direction.

I attempted to keep my speaking calendar fairly clear for the spring because I didn't know if I would be able to keep my appointments. Many occasions to speak came up out of the blue, however, and more and more of those opportunities were at churches. As had been the case at Mansfield, I had a lot more to offer my audiences than funny stories and a brief homily. I had a powerful witness to offer about how God was being glorified in my battle with cancer and I began to look forward to those opportunities like never before. Everywhere I spoke, the people were so loving and warm and welcoming. It just felt right. I knew that I was acting in God's will every time I spoke.

On the first day of May, I addressed about 600 retired educators at Callaway Gardens. I told them then that the only thing that would make me happier than speaking to retired educators was to be a retired educator. I was about to complete my thirty-eighth year in the classroom and I still didn't know if I wanted to make a career of it or not.

I had a great time with the folks at the conference. My neighbor down in Henry County, Harry Werner, had invited me and he made sure I felt right at home, including presenting me with a hug red Georgia basket full of all of my favorite things. Harry had gone through my books with a fine-toothed comb and bought me at least one of everything I had ever mentioned I liked to eat—Spam, boiled peanuts, "little Co-Colas," Vienna Sausages, Nora Mill stone-ground grits, cashew nuts—if it tasted good and was bad for you, Harry put it in that basket.

Best of all, I got to reminisce with a large group of colleagues about the good old days in education. You know the game has changed since I started school in 1958. Back then the teacher was always right; now the student seems to be. Back then the students actually had some responsibility for their own learning. Now administrators want to know what the teacher is going to do to allow a student who hasn't hit a lick at a snake all semester to pass.

When I started school it was a treat to get to go out behind the school and pound the erasers. We don't have erasers anymore, and if we did, a student couldn't be trusted to go out back of the school without fear of a lawsuit over what might happen while the student was back there.

Technology has changed, too. We used spirit masters to duplicate papers back then. You would pull the back off the paper and carefully place it on the ditto machine. There were some teachers who weren't allowed to run copies because they tended to get high on the mimeograph fluid. Now we have machines that will make 100 copies in a minute, collate, and staple pages together. We may not have paper or toner for the machines half the time, but we have the machines.

I remember the old filmstrip projectors. It was a bigger deal to be the person who advanced the filmstrip when the record player dinged than it was to be sent out to pound erasers. Now we have video streaming projected right onto giant screens and we have Magic Boards and 21st Century Classrooms. The problem is, I am still a 20th century teacher.

One thing hasn't changed, though. The relationship between the student and the teacher is still the most important component in the classroom.

Preparing for that speech in Callaway Gardens made me think about my first teacher, Miss Ruby Jordan. She was one of the most influential people in my entire life. Miss Jordan was up in years when I began my formal education in 1958. There was no kindergarten in Porterdale at that time and pre-school for four year olds hadn't been thought of, so I began my schooling in the first grade. I couldn't have had a better teacher.

Educating our children—or attempting to do so—has become a frustrating task. There are so many mandates from above—and I mean all the way to Washington, D.C.—by people who really don't understand what really goes on in the classroom that we are rapidly losing sight of the fact that the professional educator is the most valuable asset in our quest to educate and inspire the young people upon whom the future of the republic rests.

Miss Ruby Jordan was a professional in every sense of the word. She taught because she loved teaching children. Think about that for a moment. She didn't love teaching reading or writing or arithmetic—she loved teaching children and she was great at it.

Ruby Jordan understood that each child was different and that each child had different needs. She realized that everybody doesn't learn the same things at the same time in the same way. Let me give you a for-instance.

I came to the first grade already knowing how to read—like Scout Finch before me. I learned from my father while sitting in his lap at the kitchen table, peering at the pages of the Atlanta Constitution. Unlike Scout Finch's pedagogue in To Kill a Mockingbird, Miss Jordan didn't chastise me for my unorthodoxy and neither did she make me sit in a circle being bored to death with Alice and Jerry and Jip. She gave me a newspaper and assorted chapter books and made me a reading group of one. I progressed at my own pace and read about things that interested me. I still love to read, in part thanks to my father and in large part thanks to Miss Jordan's insight into my academic needs.

But she didn't just recognize my strengths. She also recognized my weaknesses, which were legion, and made sure that they were addressed as well. She didn't elevate me above other students and she didn't lower me below other students. She treated me—she treated all of us—as individuals and made sure to the best of her ability that our needs were met.

The actual knowledge she imparted to the thirty-some-odd little lintheads that were my classmates and myself was secondary to the more important life lessons she helped us learn—and there is a difference between teaching and helping someone learn. She taught us discipline. She taught us to respect ourselves and one another.

She taught us that learning could be fun. She taught us to be proud of ourselves and our parents.

It's funny what people remember. I remember that several times a year we had to fill out various forms that called for our parents' occupation. Miss Jordan taught us to put "textiles" in that form. When she had to get someone told, and from time to time all teachers have to get someone told, she would add onto her admonishment, "Put that in your pipe and smoke it."

I will never forget the day she told me that she was ashamed of me for getting in a fight, of all things. I wish I could say that I never got in another fight after that. I guess I could say it, but I'd be lying. But I haven't gotten into one since the Georgia-Missouri game in September of 2012.

Miss Ruby was great. They don't make teachers like her anymore.

I still remember my first year as a teacher. I was teaching life science to seventh graders at Cousins Middle School and I was determined to be the best teacher I could be. I was going to teach my students everything I knew. I did, too. It took me three weeks. I still had thirty-three weeks to go, so I did what a lot of teachers before and after me have done. I started reading to them from a book.

We were doing a unit on public safety and were talking about pedestrian safety. I read from a book that stated, "in New York City alone, a man gets hit by a car every fifteen minutes."

A little boy in the back of the room, Wallace Roseberry, raised his hand. Wallace was four feet high and had an afro four feet wide. This was 1974, understand. Wallace said, "Coach Huckaby, somebody ought to tell that fool to stay on the sidewalk."

That's when I first realized that what the teacher is saying and what the student is hearing isn't always the same thing.

At any rate, it was great fun being with the retired folks that May and, truth be known, for the first time I started giving a lot of thought to retiring. I didn't really want to, understand. I still enjoyed teaching and who wouldn't want to spend their days with kids as wonderful as the ones I taught. I just didn't know if I would be physically able to survive another year in the classroom.

Every time I think about retirement, I think about the legendary Erk Russell. Coach Russell was the long-time Georgia defensive coordinator under Vince Dooley who later began a dynasty at Georgia Southern University on the banks of the drainage ditch he christened "Beautiful Eagle Creek."

When Coach Russell arrived at Georgia Southern, the school didn't even have a football team. "Hell," I once heard him say, "we didn't even have a football!"

He built the team into a powerhouse and won three national championships, retiring shortly after the third. I was having breakfast with Coach Russell just a few weeks after he announced his retirement. We were at Snooky's Restaurant in Statesboro, which has recently closed its doors. I said to him, "Coach, you just won your third championship and then just walked away. You were on top of your game. How did you know it was time to quit?"

He looked at me, chomping on an unlit cigar, and said, "Huck, I'll tell you. I graduated from Auburn and got a job teaching and coaching at Grady High School. I was twenty-two years old and I don't mind telling you that some of those eighteen-year-old senior girls looked mighty good to me.

"A few years later," he continued, "I was coaching with Vince over in Athens and we had Parents' Day. I looked around and realized that a lot of the mamas were looking pretty good to me. We had Family Day at Georgia Southern last fall and I realized that the grandmamas were looking good. I knew then that it was time to quit."

Honesty compels me to admit that I have seen some pretty hot grandmamas myself lately.

Throughout the spring, I continued to hit a lot of churches: Comer United Methodist where "Bishop Bubba" is the pastor; Lawrenceville United Methodist, where Betty Faith Jaynes and her sister Peggy attend; and churches at Madison and Union Point and Athens and right here at home. Even though I had been speaking in churches for more than twenty years on a regular basis, it just started to feel more natural and more meaningful. I was beginning to see things much more clearly and I had some really good news to share. Not news about my illness, understand, but news about the power of prayer and of the saving grace of Jesus Christ.

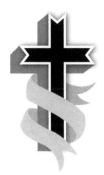

CHAPTER THIRTY

On the next to last day of May, Craig Hertwig died. There has to be a better way to hear of the passing of a dear childhood friend. My son, Jackson, texted me two simple words that night: "Sky died."

To Jackson and a generation of Athens residents and UGA students, Craig was simply "Sky." Sky was a former Georgia Bulldog and All-America tackle, former NFL lineman, local icon and bar owner who was a fixture at UGA football and basketball games.

To me, though, he will always be Craig, one of the best buddies I ever had growing up. We were in grade school and Scouts together. We played junior varsity basketball together in high school, before his family moved to Macon during his ninth grade year.

We built forts and played with army men and got in all kinds of trouble. After three years apart in high school, we were reunited at UGA when we both moved into McWhorter Hall—he as a football player and I as a basketball manager.

Craig's mother, Merritt, was our Cub Scout den mother. Listening to her talk about politics and her two "daughters with the car," Merry and Willa, was as much fun as learning to make crafts and drink Kool-Aid and whatever else we did as Wolf Cubs.

Ironically, Craig was a Georgia Tech fan because his brother, Ed, had played at Tech before transferring to South Carolina. Craig kept a Tech helmet in his bedroom—the one his brother had worn against the Georgia Bullpups in the Thanksgiving Day Freshman Classic at

Historic Grant Field. Every year, Craig and I would bet a "big Co-Cola" on the outcome of the Tech-Georgia varsity game. I bought a lot of Cokes for a while, but then Vince Dooley was hired at Georgia and I was on the drinking end of the soda exchange.

Neatness was never a priority for Craig. He played hard at recess and usually came back to class with his shirt tail out and a little dirt on his face. I remember hearing our fourth-grade teacher, Mrs. Betty Robertson, complaining to Craig's mama about his appearance. She told Mrs. Betty, "If you'll just teach him enough math to get in Georgia Tech, I'll worry about how Craig looks and dresses."

Craig had lived in Macon before moving to Porterdale and was the only one in our class who had been taught to say "isn't" instead of "ain't." I was delighted to learn when our paths crossed in college that he had unlearned most of his proper grammar along the way.

During our first Boy Scout encampment at Bert Adams, Craig and I earned the ire of our Scoutmaster, Boonie Barnes, by putting out the campfire one night the way Tenderfoot Scouts have been putting out campfires for years. We had to run to the lake and back six times.

Porterdale kids were very creative and would find all sorts of ways to make our own fun during the summer. We would play marathon games of Monopoly that would last for weeks, and when we would choose up sides to play army, some of our battles were as drawn out as the Battle of the Bulge. Usually it was the younger kids—those the ages of Craig and me—against the older kids. We would get trounced, but one day Craig decided that we would get the high ground and win the day. The highest thing in Porterdale was the water tower—so we climbed it. We did, indeed, win the day. It was well worth the whippings we got when our parents found out.

Another time, when Craig's parents were supposedly gone for the day, we wound up in a water balloon fight against the big kids. We ran into Craig's empty house, where we thought we would be safe. Randy Digby, Steve Piper, and Phil Shaw followed us right into the house—all three throwing balloons with both hands. Craig's parents drove up at a most inopportune time. More whippings.

His dad, Big Ed, made it up to us though by taking Craig and me to the first baseball game ever played in Atlanta Stadium. It was a night I will never forget.

The last time I saw Craig was in the winter of 2011. I was speaking at a church in Hart County and stopped in the Nowhere Bar to say hello. I ordered a Coke and the young bartender looked very nervous. He said, "Mister, Sky doesn't like people to wear ties in here."

"I'm glad you mentioned Sky," I told him. "That's who I'm looking for. I'm here to whip his tail."

The bartender said, "Sir, are you crazy?"

I said, "Get him in here!" So he did.

Craig came flying in the door, looking around to see who his combatant would be. When he saw me at the bar, he laughed and had a Coke with me. We talked about Georgia football and old times, but if I had known it would be the last time we would be together, I swear I would have thought of something better to say than, "See you soon."

But that is what I did say and now Jackson had texted me that he was, quite unexpectedly, dead. It seems that Craig had been playing cards with his buddies the previous Monday night—it might have been a Tuesday—and complained of not feeling well. The next day he went to see his doctor, who found an irregular heartbeat and sent him to the hospital. It is my understanding that he drove himself there. His condition steadily worsened and by Wednesday evening, this gentle giant of a man was dead. The news hit me especially hard because I had been spending so much time contemplating the possibility of my own death.

Here is where the God-instances started. Jerry Varnado was the chaplain on call at St. Mary's Hospital in Athens the night Craig died. Lisa and I had met Jerry and his wife, Beverly, a couple of years earlier. We were all at UGA freshman orientation with our children. Jerry, like me, married way up, by the way. Our paths had not crossed since, but Beverly had recently published her first book, a Christian novel set on St. Simons Island. Having read in my columns over the years how much we enjoyed spring break on the Georgia Coast, she sent me a copy in the mail just before our first trip to Houston. Her book brought great comfort to Lisa and me.

Here is where things got a bit strange. Jerry, before becoming a lawyer, which preceded him becoming a Methodist minister, had played football at Georgia and had coached on Vince Dooley's staff. He had been Craig Hertwig's freshman football coach—and had not seen him much since. Craig owned a bar, as I said. He didn't go to church, so, as Jerry said, "He didn't frequent my establishment and I didn't frequent his."

Jerry only served as chaplain one night every three months—or four times a year. He was shocked to find out when he was called to the hospital that the family he was coming to comfort was that of his favorite player. Jerry remembered having read in one of my columns that Craig and I were boyhood friends and neighbors, so he called me at home the night after Sky died to try and glean some material for the funeral service he had been asked to preach. After we talked for a while, Jerry asked me if I would do the eulogy at the service. Of course, I was most honored to do so.

The chapel was overflowing for the service. I was reunited with Craig's siblings, Merry and Ed and Bootsie, none of whom I had seen in years. It felt right for me to be there with them in their time of grief, and as Jerry said, "The service could not have gone better."

As I drove home that afternoon, I had a lot of time to ponder the events of the past two months and I came to realize that when you sincerely ask God to lead you in the path He would have you to go, God will lead you in the path He would have you to go, so you'd better be ready. For once in my life, I was. I truly was.

When you have cancer, you need a safe place to go—or a couple of them. By that I mean you need somewhere to go where you can get away from your cares and worries and just be. It is OK if people are around—in fact, it is a good thing for people to be around, as long as they are people who will talk to you, and, more importantly, listen to you if you want to talk or be listened to, but who will leave you alone and let you be if you don't.

I have had two such bunkers during my battle. One is Evans Market in the Magnet community of south Rockdale County. Ben Evans, and his wife, Dolores, have been in the produce business for about thirty years and I have been buying produce and pumpkins and Christmas trees from them for about thirty years. A while back, though—and I can't say exactly when or how it happened, it just did—the Evans family and I began to develop a much closer relationship than just customer and 'mater man. We have become very close friends and if I don't show up at his place of business by ten o'clock Saturday mornings, he begins to worry. If I am not there by noon, he is apt to pick up his phone and call me to find out why.

Many an afternoon, during the worst part of my illness, when I had nowhere else to go, I would get in my car and drive down to Ben's. I would usually sit in one of the two rocking chairs on his porch that he painted red on my behalf. Ben could always sense if I wanted to be engaged in conversation or if I just wanted to sit. That's a rare quality for a human being to possess. He always reminded me that everyone in his church, Salem Baptist in Stockbridge, was praying for me. He needn't have, though. Scarcely a day went by for months that I didn't receive a note or a prayer-gram from Dolores or one of her friends. Every one was appreciated and every one lifted my spirits and reminded me to thank the good Lord for friends like the Evans family.

Ben would also let me know about the dozens and dozens of his customers that stopped in and asked about me each week. Ben will never know how much his friendship, concern, and prayers have truly meant to me, no matter how many times I tell him. But I still say that he is terrible at math.

My other safe haven has been Henderson's restaurant on Highway 36, south of Covington.

I started eating catfish at Clarence Henderson's when I was a child and I haven't slowed up since. Henderson's is truly a family restaurant, owned and operated by the Henderson family, and for years they have made me feel like part of that family. At any low point in my life, going to Henderson's for a bite of catfish, coleslaw, hushpuppies, and sweet tea has made me feel better—and as good as the food is, it is the Henderson family that I really keep going back for.

About the same time I was diagnosed with cancer, David Henderson was too. David is the oldest brother in the family and is an attorney by day and the world's best catfish cook by night. We have already lost his younger brother, Clarence, to cancer. David is putting up a valiant fight. He has undergone surgery at Emory to remove a lung and has endured I don't know how many rounds of chemo-therapy. Even so, I can still find him at the restaurant, frying up the delicious food that screams, "I love the American South" at me every time I walk through the door of the establishment.

As tough a go as David was having, his mother, Frances, and his sisters, Deborah, Clarice, and Mary Anne, always had time to check in on me and I know that their prayers on my behalf have never waned. Deborah is my biggest promoter and openly chastises people on Facebook if they haven't read my latest column or bought my latest book. As with the Evans', I love and respect the Hender-son family more than I can say. Both those families are examples of what made America great. Honest, unpretentious, hard-working, God-fearing folks who are not afraid to get their hands dirty or work up a sweat. I wish I knew more folks like them.

I am thankful to have folks like that praying for me every day.

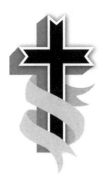

CHAPTER THIRTY ONE

I won't say which grandmother inspired me, but I did retire at the end of the school year.

It didn't work out, though, and I went back to the school in the fall—half time, which was always the plan if it turned out that I was able, and I was.

As much as I enjoy teaching and as much as I love Heritage High School, being out of school was one of the best things that could have happened at the particular time it did. I needed rest, and I was finally able to get some.

I started sleeping in every morning. Some days I didn't get up before 6:30. Jackson, who had just graduated with his master's degree from UGA, moved back home to spend time with me and eat a summer's worth of home cooking. Jenna left for her six-week mission in Africa and I missed her mightily. Jamie was still being Jamie, selling drugs, taking care of the folks who came into the pharmacy, and wondering if and when her boyfriend, Chris Fairchild, was going to pop the question. It was a good summer and I could feel myself getting stronger.

My one downfall of the season, however, was picking up a horrible and expensive addiction—golf.

Mark Twain called golf "a good walk spoiled." He was wrong in my case. I don't walk, I ride in the cart, and I am terrible at the game. But if I can be out on the links with Jackson or my buddy

Mark, the score doesn't really matter because the companionship is more important.

Not that I don't want to get better, understand. I am still the fierce competitor that my friend, Bonham Johnson, reminds me I was back in the day. I have even bought Ben Hogan's book on how to play the game and have taken up going to the driving range to practice. But golf took up a lot of my time—and my money—during the summer. I had to have something to do during those twelve weeks between visits to M.D. Anderson. And, as I said, despite playing too much golf and because of extra rest, I did begin to feel stronger. I walked a couple of miles every morning and would have eaten a lot better—if I could have resisted the temptation to join a cult.

Let me explain. I am an Egghead. My name is Darrell and I own a Big Green Egg and I cannot stop cooking on it.

Remember back when there was a Circuit City electronics store in our area? They ran a particular commercial for years. A father and his son would visit Circuit City over and over and over, gazing wistfully at the widescreen high-definition television that they hoped to buy and bring to their own home one day. They would return with each passing season and take up residence in front of the TV set until the store closed and they had to go home to their own antique 35-inch set.

That's me, except I yearned for a Big Green Egg. For years I have found every excuse in the world to drop by Cowan Ace Hardware for this and that. As often as I visited Cowan's, one would think that I would have the neatest yard and most squared away home in the area. One would be wrong. My numerous trips to the hardware store were actually thinly veiled excuses to visit the grill section and stare at the Eggs, dreaming of the day that I could own one myself.

For the uninitiated, a Big Green Egg is a unique type of ceramic grill, smoker, roaster, oven and all-round cooking device perfected by Georgian Ed Fisher in the 1970s. The first person I ever knew who owned one was former Ebenezer UMC pastor Davis Hancock. He used to rave about how efficiently they cooked and what delicious and moist food they produced. Back in those days, the product was mostly promoted through small ads in the sports pages of the big city newspaper—often right next to those for Asian massage parlors.

As the years passed, more and more folks I knew became Egg converts and for the past five or six years, one of the hot topics of conversation at school—especially when Bob Bradley and Casey Teal get together—has been that same smoker. Bob and Casey would compare cooking techniques, citing cook times and temperatures as if they were quoting passages from Deuteronomy, and the conversation was always laced with talks of rubs and spices and marinades and what sort of wood chips created the best flavor.

Now understand, these weren't casual conversations or words shared in passing. These were long passionate discussions. It was obvious that these guys were committed to what they were doing.

But talk is cheap. The proof is in the pudding—or, in this case, the ribs, Boston Butt, and smoked turkey breast. I had the opportunity to sample some of Casey's cooking at an Athens tailgate party one October. A couple of years later, Bob Bradley held court with a wide array of his food at the Georgia-Colorado game. Last fall, he offered samples of his wares at Cowan's while I signed copies of my new cookbook. When he produced a smoked turkey for me last Thanksgiving that my own kids said was better than anything I had ever cooked, my mind was made up. I would own a Big Green Egg.

I finally pulled the trigger and I am here to tell you that my life has been changed. I was already interested in becoming an Egghead. Now I am committed to being one. I simply cannot stop cooking on my Egg.

How do I love thee? Let me count the ways. For one thing it uses lump charcoal, which starts quickly, without lighter fluid, and burns consistently. I can get my cooker to a set temperature and it will stay there for hours. I'm talking ten or twelve hours. I ain't making this up, y'all. The coal burns with very little ash and what doesn't burn up can be reused.

The dome shape of the cooker and the thick ceramic sides hold in heat and flavor and moisture like nothing I've ever experienced—and, no—I am not an official spokesman for the company. So far I have cooked Boston Butt twice, ribs three times, whole chickens a half-dozen times, and smoked turkey. I have also cooked some of the best steaks I have ever eaten—600 degrees, four minutes to the side.

Every bite of food has been delicious and, besides all that, it is just a lot of fun to experiment with rubs and spices and marinades and, well, all those things I've listened to Bob and Casey talk about for years. Plus I got a huge compliment from my kids when they said, "Daddy, your stuff is just as good as Bob's!" That alone was worth the price.

Is there a downside to the Big Green Egg? Oh, absolutely. I am eating way too much meat and have gained twelve pounds—but they are a happy twelve pounds.

Lisa and I also went on a cruise this summer. Our friends, Clay and Holle Stapp, were going on one to celebrate their thirtieth wedding anniversary. Since ours was coming up and since the Stapps had been gung-ho enough to brave the wilds of Jekyll Island hunting wild boar with us, not to mention dodging bears and Mexican bandits along the Rio Grande, we thought the least we could do was tour the Caribbean with them.

Let me tell you what it was like. There was water, water everywhere, but nary a drop to drink. That wasn't a problem, though, because there was plenty of other stuff—and don't even get me started on what there was to eat.

We had a grand time checking out Christopher Columbus's old stomping grounds. Now that was a brave dude. He set his stern to Europe and his bow toward the setting sun and did what no one had ever done before—at least no one who actually documented his feats. He sailed west across the Atlantic Ocean and didn't stop until he found land. They didn't call him Admiral of the Ocean Seas for nothing, you know.

Nowadays, Christopher Columbus is vilified because he kidnapped some of the natives he found on the islands he explored and took them back to Spain for show-and-tell. Folks say that Columbus didn't know where he was going or where he had been and that he didn't discover America because the Vikings may or may not have been here first. Plus Columbus' men and those who would follow introduced the Indians to diseases for which they had no immunities and forced Christianity on them and, well, you know all about that. You can blame all the evils of modern society on either Christopher Columbus or George W. Bush.

I still say Columbus was a brave man and he opened the door to a whole new world. If you are going to blame death and disease and destruction on Columbus, it seems like you'd have to give him a little credit for Coca-Cola, the space program, defeating Hitler and Tojo, and winning the Cold War, too.

But I digress—as usual.

I thought the cruise would be right down my alley. Usually when I take a vacation, it takes me a week or two to recover. I'm not what you would call a stationary person. I will drive a hundred miles out of the way to take a picture of the world's largest—or even third largest—ball of string or roll of aluminum foil. I also have a genetic disorder that prevents me from driving past a historical marker. I have never bypassed a scenic overlook without stopping, and if somebody—anybody—tells me there is something to do or see within a day's drive of my destination, I am going to make sure I do it or see it.

Vacations, Huckaby-style, are exhausting, understand. But this time, I could not afford to be exhausted. I couldn't afford a vacation, either, but that is another story for another day.

Now this wasn't my first rodeo—or my first cruise. Sixty-five stalwart souls accompanied me on an inner-passage adventure in Alaska a few years back and my kids let me accompany them on a cruise with the high school band one year. But I didn't have a great amount of experience with cruising.

This one worked out great for a while, but being me, I overdid it. I tried to eat everything there was to eat and it probably wasn't a real good idea to climb Dunn River Falls in Jamaica. I wound up hurting all over and could barely able to walk by the end of the week. I also got sick and could no longer eat and lost ten pounds. It was worth it, though, if for no other reason than because of what happened on Grand Cayman Island in the middle of the trip.

It happened on a Thursday. I was about to board a boat on Grand Cayman Island to have a go at swimming with the stingrays. Right in front of me in line was Roger Mayhart, a seed salesman from Bogart, Georgia. It turns out that he works for Pennington Seed, a company started by the late Brooks Pennington, who used to be my state senator.

I didn't know any of this at the time, of course. I had never met Roger and had no idea who he was. As it turns out, he reads my column and recognized me somehow from the fifteen-year-old picture the papers still run with it. He turned to me in line and said, "I just want you to know that my family and I are praying for you."

Let me tell you something. It is indeed heartening to have total stranger walk up to you in a foreign country and tell you that he is praying for you.

Roger was with his two beautiful daughters, Laura, who is a senior at Clemson, bless her heart, and Leah, who will be started school in August at the University of Georgia, hallowed be thy name. We had a long conversation about what was grander than the Cayman Islands themselves and found that we have a lot in common. I hope our paths cross again soon. At any rate, he warmed my heart that day and, once again reminded me that there are no coincidences out there—only God-incidences.

It did take me about two weeks to recover from my cruise vacation. That was good timing, though, because I was feeling better just in time for my return trip to M.D. Anderson.

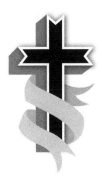

CHAPTER THIRTY TWO

I was pretty sure I would only have to stay two days in Houston on the second trip, so I made plans to fly out—alone. I had to be a big boy sometime, and besides, plane tickets are expensive and Lisa needed to stay home and work anyway. The trip was seamless. I got into Hobby Airport around three and caught the shuttle to the hotel. They had my room ready, and since Lisa wasn't with me, I did not have to take a second tour of the hospital district. I did ride the Rotary shuttle to Pappas, however, for some Texas brisket. It's what they consider barbecue out there. Then I came "home" to the hotel, spent a little time in the pool, and then listened to the Elvis imitator that came by to entertain in the lobby.

They have something special for the patients every evening. It's a great place, y'all.

I couldn't wait for the nurse to take my blood the next morning and then I couldn't wait to get back that afternoon to see the doctor for the results. He had told me earlier that I should hope for my PSA to get down around 2.4, but not to be disappointed if it were a little higher.

I was not disappointed. The next afternoon, Dr. Pagliaro rolled in with a big smile on his face. "Congratulations," he said. "Your PSA is undetectable."

"Undetectable?" I stammered quizzically.

"Yep," he responded. "It is less than 0.0. Undetectable."

"What does that mean," I asked.

"It means that we give you another treatment and I'll see you in twelve weeks," he said.

"Is my cancer gone?" I marveled.

"It will never be gone," the doctor assured me. "It is still in your bones so we will still have to give you treatments, but the PSA is undetectable at the time, and that is good."

So is God, all the time.

I picked up my bags and headed to the airport. I could probably have flown home without a plane. I couldn't wait to tell Lisa. I couldn't wait to tell the kids. I couldn't wait to tell my sister, Myron. I couldn't wait to tell the world. So I didn't. I called all of the above—except the world, of course. To take care of telling the world, I posted on Facebook and then sat down in the airport lobby. While I waited for my plane to board, I wrote the following column:

One is the Loneliest Number; Zero is the Best

I was reading about Elvis last week—I know he's been dead since 1977, but I can still read about him can't I?

According to the article I was reading, Elvis was big into numerology. One of his favorite books supposedly was Cheiro's Book of Numbers, which was said to explain the occult significance between numbers and human events.

Now I don't believe in any of that, but there have always been certain numbers that have held great meaning for me. Lots of us have favorite numbers, don't you know.

Three is a good one. I have three children and that has worked out pretty well so far. Three is the number of the trinity, too. "The three men I admire the most—the Father, Son and Holy Ghost—they took the first train for the coast . . ."

The great Babe Ruth wore number 3. One of my favorite baseball stories is the one Jim Bouton tells about reporting to spring training for his rookie season with the Yankees. Unhappy with the astronomically high number he was given, he asked for a lower one. Told that his 66, or whatever number he'd been given, was the lowest available, Bouton replied, "I didn't see anybody wearing number 3 out there."

Gotta love his brass.

Seven has always been one of my favorite numbers, too. Unlike Seinfeld's George Costanza, I never wanted to name one of my kids 7, but Mickey Mantle did wear it and Mickey Mantle was my hero.

Of course we can't talk about uniform numbers without mentioning 34, which is the Holy Grail for those of the red and black persuasion. If I ever have to choose a number between 1 and 100—or infinity—you can bet your bippy I am picking 34. And if I ever have an occasion to play roulette—which I've yet to do in my first sixty years on the planet—I will put whatever money I have to lose—which won't be much—on 34 and let it ride.

They say that confession is good for the soul and my soul can always use a boost, so I will make a confession that will make me look really silly in the eyes of many. When I am able, I like to swim for exercise. A couple of summers ago I was swimming a mile every day. Jack Bauerle would have been proud.

At my home pool, a mile is a little more than 34 laps—see how numbers connect?—and let's face it, after a few laps the numbers start running together. Did I just finish ten laps or did I just finish twelve? To keep up with my laps I would assign the number of one of my favorite athletes to each lap. When I finished lap three I would say to myself, "Babe Ruth." When I finished lap nineteen I would say "Johnny Unitas" and when I finished lap twenty-four I would say "Willie Mays." When I got to Herschel I was done. Laugh if you will, but it worked.

Not all significant numbers in my life are jersey numbers, of course. For me, 412 used to be a big one because it was the number of our mailbox at the Porterdale Post Office. For years my address was P.O. Box 412, Porterdale. Ironically, when I moved into the now-defunct McWhorter Hall at UGA, my room number was 412 and my mailing address became Box 412, McWhorter Hall, Athens.

Elvis might have been on to something, come to think of it.

One hundred twenty-nine has been a special number since that night in 1967 when Wills High School beat the Newton Rams, ending our world record home court basketball winning streak at 129. My mind recognizes that number wherever it appears. There can be clocks everywhere and I will never notice if it is 2:10 or 3:47 or 1:19—but when that sucker hits 1:29, my eyes will take notice.

Another significant number in my life is 7060 because that was my parents' phone number for four decades—with various prefixes and area codes added as the years went by and the phone company grew. The number 1218 stands out, too, because it is my anniversary. I didn't know what happiness was until I got married. Then it was too late.

I told you all of that to tell you this. I have a brand new favorite number and I think it will remain my favorite number for a long, long time.

That number is 0, y'all, and not because some ball player wears it on his uniform. 0 is the level of Prostate-specific antigen the doctors at M.D. Anderson found in my blood last week. That is significant because for the past fifteen months, through surgery and radiation and all sorts of horrible medications, my PSA had been rising exponentially with each and every blood test.

My doctor said he has no explanation for the sudden extreme drop to "non-detectable."

But I do, y'all. I do. Thanks—and please keep them coming.

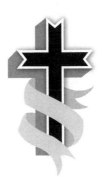

CHAPTER THIRTY THREE

God was keeping me busy as Independence Day approached. I had received many, many invitations to speak at area churches. They weren't just for senior banquets or Wednesday night suppers, either. I was being inviting to address Sunday night services and to even bring the message on Sunday morning at a couple of churches. I was blown away by the invitations and the response of the congregations I addressed.

Jerry Varnado, my friend with whom I had presided over Craig Hertwig's funeral, invited me to deliver the homecoming message at his church, Ray's United Methodist in Bishop. I received invitations to teach classes and to speak at special services at Conyers First United Methodist, where I had already presented several sermons that year. It was actually all a bit bewildering, but that's just because I was looking at the world through my eyes, not God's.

A couple of days after the Fourth of July, we all packed up and headed back to Salem for camp meeting. What a difference a year can make. The previous year at Salem, I had been so scared and so emotional and so sick. This year, I felt great and was at perfect peace and didn't have a worry in the world. Jenna was safely home from Africa, Jackson and his girlfriend, Brittney, whose relationship had begun as a Salem romance two years earlier, were there and so was Jamie and, for at least part of the week, her soon-to-be fiancé, Chris. Life was good.

YEA THOUGH I WALK

My mother-in-law, Bitzi, and her sister, Renee, kept a lot of good food on the table; Jackson kept a lot of homemade peach ice cream on the ready after evening services; and we had a grand week of worship and celebration. Scott and Mary Anne Gordon, two of my dearest friends in the world, made it out several times. I love spending time with Scott and Mary Anne. They make me want to be a better person, and I would say that even if Mary Anne didn't make the best scuppernong jelly in the world—but she does, and she is always good to share.

The previous year, I had hibernated in my bedroom most of the week. This year, I got to spend lots of time visiting with my Salem friends. Daniel Farley and I solved most of the world's problems around the long kitchen table in the back room of our "tent." I got to visit with his wife, Paige, one of my very favorite people in the whole world, a few times, too. Ken "Barbie" Parkinson came by every night to offer his words of wisdom and so did Joe Cook, world's coolest person. Life was good at Salem. Life was very good.

I taught an adult class on "Jesus' Bucket List," and had about seventy folks there every day, which made me feel good. We spent our week learning about Jesus' last week on earth.

Of course, Sam Ramsey presided over the week as he has for the past umpteen years. Sam has been a close friend and confidant for a lot of years. My first job was helping Sam deliver furniture when I was fourteen and he has contributed more to the promotion and success of Salem Camp Meeting than any person I know that has contributed to any institution. And, yes, his wife, Becky, and her identical twin sister, Alice, played the twin grand pianos three services a day.

Life was almost back to normal at Salem. Almost, with one major difference. Every morning and every night I could feel God working in my life. He talked to me through the hymns and especially through the words of the Methodist preacher of the week, Winston Worrel.

I have to say here that church services for me are sometimes like a spectator sport. I love the music—especially the old gospel hymns—and I love critiquing the preachers, although I probably shouldn't have told that. We have had lots of memorable preachers at Salem, although some are memorable for better reasons than others.

Charles Sineath was one of my favorites. Charles Sineath once told a story about his barber shop closing and having to get his hair cut at a "beauty salon." He said, "I'd rather be caught coming out of a liquor store than a beauty salon.

Gil Watson is another of my favorites. He is one of the world's great story tellers and if you ever get a chance to hear him tell about his first deep water baptism in the pond behind the little country church he served, don't pass it up. Gil has been known to dress up as Joel Chandler Harris and tell an Uncle Remus story or two. I am pretty good with the Tar Baby and the Laughing Place, myself, so I like that about Gil.

Gil Watson delivered one of the best lines I have ever heard when Gov. Sonny Perdue invited him to be one of the speakers on the steps of the Georgia State Capitol when we gathered a few years back to pray for rain. Gil chastised the crowd by saying, "We are all here to pray for rain," and then, holding up his, said, "and I'm the only one who brought my umbrella."

Dennis Kinlaw was one of the most amazing theologians I ever heard. He is the resident genius at Ashbury College and would lean across the pulpit and stare you right in the face. You felt like you were getting the message right from God. Probably because you were, in a way.

There have been so many great ones at Salem. Bishop Bevel Jones; my own pastor, John Beyers, who wishes he were John Wesley; Phil DeMore, who goes back with me to my high school days; Jonathan Holston, himself now a bishop; and of course, John Ed Matheson, of Montgomery, Alabama. John Ed is one of my all-time favorites. He ate more of Jackson's peach ice cream in one week than Joe Cook and Daniel Farley put together. He also told the story one night about Simon Peter stepping out of the boat and walking on water to meet Jesus, and added, "not even Bear Bryant had done it at that time."

The list goes on and on and on. I even heard the legendary Bishop Arthur Moore preach under that tabernacle.

The favorite Salem preacher emeritus, however, has to be now and forevermore, the Baptist minister Marshall Edwards. I think he has preached at Salem seven times, but it could be twelve. I have lost count. I just know that every time he comes, the tabernacle is full and he blesses my heart. Marshall and I are close friends, and I was reminded recently that I have to give back the prayers I am receiving. When I heard the distressing news that he had suffered a heart attack at his home in Blowing Rock, N.C., I wore out the knees of three pairs of overalls praying for Marshall, and as of this writing, the prayers have worked. He is doing well.

Marshall says that every song can become a hymn by singing "amen" at the end, and I have heard him prove it a time or two by adding "amen" to Zip-A-Dee-Doo-Dah.

Marshall preaches—and lives—love more than he does hellfire and brimstone and makes his sermons personal by telling stories about his family. Some of them may even be true. My favorite Marshall story is the one he tells on himself, about when he was a student at Baylor and dating his then-girlfriend, now-wife, Doris Dillard.

Apparently, Marshall hadn't been quick enough to make his intentions toward Doris known and she received an invitation to attend a Texas A&M football game with a member of the Aggie Corps of Cadets. Marshall found out that those Aggies kiss their dates after every touchdown and on this particular day, A&M beat some hapless opponent 72-0. Needless to say, Marshall had a miserable afternoon. The next day, however, he showed up at Doris Dillard's home with a bouquet of eleven red roses and a card that read—are you ready for this?—"You are the twelfth." The rest, as they say, is history.

The first Friday of camp meeting this year, I went down to the tabernacle in the early afternoon, before too many people were around, just to sit and meditate. As I sat there, I found myself laughing out loud as I remembered a particular Saturday night way back when I was still in college. I was at the service alone—I went to Georgia, you recall, and not many of my friends spent their Saturday nights in church. I forget who the preacher was that night, but he got on a roll and was really shelling down the corn. At the end of his sermon he gave a powerful altar call.

That preacher urged everyone in the congregation to think about the one sin that they struggled with the most. Then he asked us all to walk down that sawdust aisle and lay our one sin at the altar and pray over it. He promised that our sin, whatever it was, would be picked up by Jesus and taken away forever.

I was a typical twenty-one year-old, in most ways, and I found myself having lustful thoughts quite often. These thoughts made me feel guilty—and this was before Jimmy Carter reminded us in the pages of Playboy that lustful thoughts were just as bad as doing the deed. Jesus had already let us know that, but Jimmy Earl hadn't.

I was convicted to get up and walk down the aisle and lay lust upon the Salem altar. I did, too. I prayed earnestly and reverently that I would never be tempted by lust again, and I was convinced that I wouldn't be. When I finished praying, I just stepped back and took a seat on the front pew and continued to pray.

While I was praying in the pew, a girl I had known all my life decided to come down and lay her sins at the altar, too. She shall remain nameless here, but she was about six feet tall with thick red hair and had the longest legs and was wearing the shortest miniskirt I had ever seen. When I lifted my eyes after I had finished praying she was kneeling right in front of me.

That's the first time I understood what Voltaire meant when he wrote, "God is a comedian, playing to an audience that is afraid to laugh."

I knew then I was in for a good week.

Once Taps had been played each night, I turned in and then lay awake, much as I had the previous summer, but for a different reason. The previous summer, I lay awake wondering if my life were about to come to an end. This summer I was convinced that it was going to continue for a long, long while. I was a bit like John Wesley, who was advised during a low point in his early ministry, "Preach faith until you have it." I had pronounced my assurance of healing until I had experienced it.

I had believed that God would spare me, at least for a while longer. I had learned over the previous fifteen months that every day is truly a gift from God and I was determined that I would not squander that gift—not for a second longer. I wanted to be sure that I lived my life in accordance with His plan for my life—and my prayer all week at Salem was that He would show me, with clarity, what that plan was.

In reality, of course, I knew—and had known for quite some time.

When I was growing up in Julia A. Porter Methodist Church—I think it was "Memorial" back then, not "United," I was always enamored of our preachers. Preacher Dillard was the first one I can recall. I thought he was as old as God, but now that I am old, I realize he could have been anywhere from thirty-five to seventy-five.

They tell me that when I was about two-and-a-half years old, everyone had gathered in the downstairs fellowship hall of our church for a fifth Sunday covered dish dinner. Someone asked the preacher to say grace. I was hungry, my mama's fried chicken and deviled eggs were on the table, and all I heard was offer thanks. I stood up to the table and said the only meal-time prayer I knew when I was two. I said, "Ask the blessing, ask the blessing, ask the blessing, Amen!"

Everyone laughed, like everyone does when something like that happens, and then someone told the preacher to pray again.

Again, I took a step forward and said, "Ask the blessing, ask the blessing, ask the blessing, Amen!"

After I delivered that same blessing for the third time, Preacher Dillard said, "That's good enough!" and we all ate dinner.

Preacher Peters was another preacher I remember. I know that he was younger than Preacher Dillard because his hair was black instead of white and his wife was pregnant while he was here—except nobody ever said the word "pregnant" in those days, not in mixed company. They said expecting or, at the very worst, "PG."

The main thing I remember about Preacher Peter's time at Porterdale was how everybody laughed at me when I came home from church one day and excitedly announced that the preacher's wife was wearing a "baby dress," which is what I assumed a maternity outfit was called.

One of my favorite preachers of all time was A.J. "Gus" Bruyere. He was from Green Bay, Wisconsin, and might have been the first

Yankee I ever knew. I know he was the first person I ever knew who preferred professional football to college football. His daddy had played for the original Green Bay Packers—or maybe it was his grandfather—but he had a model of Lambeau Field on a desk in his office and I loved to go in every Sunday and gaze at it.

Preacher Bruyere was a different sort than most of the preachers we had known at Julia A. Porter. Instead of a dark suit, he preached in a black robe with different colored stoles for the different liturgical seasons. I was really curious about everything that went on at church and would always sit by my daddy and ask him about everything.

I will never forget the first time Gus Bruyere served communion. In the past when we celebrated the Lord's Supper, Blackie Jeffries and Jake Hunt and some of them would crumble up some soda crackers in the communion plates and pour a little Welch's grape juice into those little shot glasses and we would nibble on a cracker and drink a sip of juice.

That's not how Preacher Gus did it. He stood at the altar and held up a long loaf of freshly baked bread—my daddy said Gus would have preferred to have been a Catholic priest if it hadn't been for that whole celibacy thing—and said words over it. I whispered to my daddy, "What does that mean? What does it mean when he does that?"

Daddy told me, "That means that the bread represents the body of Christ and that it was broken for you and me."

Then the preacher held up a big silver chalice and poured grape juice into it from another fancy bottle.

"What does that mean?" I asked. "Why is he doing that?"

"That means that the wine represents the blood of Christ and that it was shed for you and me."

Every Sunday before he preached, Reverend Bruyere would take off his watch and place it on the pulpit so he could keep his eye on it. "What does that mean?" I would ask. "What does it mean when he does that?"

My daddy would sadly shake his head and say, "It doesn't mean a thing. It doesn't mean a cotton picking thing."

One of my favorite Porterdale ministers was Harold Lyda, who is a dear, dear man with the gentlest spirit of anyone I had ever known.

Reverend Lyda was the pastor brought me into full membership of the church. He was the pastor who oversaw my Eagle Scout project. He was the pastor who came to visit me every day when I almost died while a freshman in college.

Reverend Lyda happened to come to Porterdale during my teenage years, and you know how teenagers are. Bill Cosby's stories about growing up in Philadelphia were very popular on eight-track tapes back then. Oh, hush. You already knew I was old. All of my friends and I listened to Cosby's stories about Fat Albert and his friends, one of which was known as "Old Weird Harold," who was so tall and thin that they used to stick chewing gum on his head and use him to get baseballs out of the sewers.

Unfortunately, the good reverend was very tall and very thin, so naturally we called him "Old Weird Harold," although he was neither old nor weird. What he was was—and is—is a very dear man.

Preacher Lyda had been in the Navy during World War II. During one of his visits to our house, Daddy learned that the preacher had been in the Philippines when the notorious typhoon had come through. I asked him if he were scared. He told me that he wasn't sacred at all. He said he knew it was coming and asked one of his buddies to lash him to his cot. Then he said his prayers, went to sleep, and slept right through it.

If anyone else, including most preachers I know, had told me that story, I would not have believed it. When Harold Lyda told It, I didn't doubt it for a second.

I have always enjoyed being around preachers, you see—and still do. I enjoy talking to them. I enjoy listening to some of them and I enjoy studying their craft. Preachers have to have a lot of the skills—or gifts, if you will—that I have. They have to be good with words. They have to be comfortable around people. Good ones have to be good story-tellers. Fruitful ones have to love Jesus Christ and understand the Bible and be called to proclaim the gospel of Christ to a lost world.

I have realized that all of those qualifications suit me to a tee—and have for a long, long time. Yes, I am saying what you think I am saying. I have been called to preach the gospel of Jesus Christ since

230

I was a teenager and I have intentionally avoided that call—out of fear, out of stubbornness—because I have always wanted to do what I want to do, for reasons I can't begin to explain.

I have felt guilty about ignoring that call for a long time, too, which may explain a good deal of my orneriness.

Mrs. Dora Ivey was the first person to recognize that call in me. I was in high school, maybe the eleventh grade, and we were in Sunday school one day. All the youth used to meet together for singing and prayers and then we would go into separate rooms with people our own age to study the lesson. You'd better not miss, either, or Mrs. Dora would get onto you when you came into White's, where she worked, to buy new underwear or look at the fishing lures.

We were gathered together before we split up and Mrs. Ivey said, completely out of the blue, God told me that somebody in this room is going to make a preacher. Everyone in the room grinned and looked at Tony Allison, who had dropped out of high school and joined the Army. Tony gave God credit for allowing him to survive a year in Vietnam and had been giving his testimony every chance he got. "It's Tony, isn't it?" every kid in the room asked.

Every kid in the room, that is, except me. I knew exactly who Mrs. Dora Ivey was talking about because God had told me the exact same thing—and I knew that it was me that God was calling.

"No," she said, "Shaking her head. It's not Tony." Her eyes locked on mine. Thankfully nobody else noticed, but I knew. What is worse, God knew that I knew.

I toyed with the notion. I did. I spoke at church on Youth Sunday and gave my own testimony at different churches from time to time. I always spoke highly of God and Jesus. I was good. I didn't drink or smoke and didn't cuss as much as some I knew. I even talked about preaching with some of my close friends. Terri Hubbard and I had plans at one time to form an evangelism team. She would sing and I would regale audiences worldwide with my charm and charisma and we would all sing, Kumbaya and live happily ever after. Terri and I have never gotten around to doing that—at least not yet.

When I was a senior in college and about to receive my education degree, I decided that I just couldn't run away from the call to preach any longer. I went to our pastor at Porterdale and told him that I wanted to attend seminary; I wanted to make a preacher.

He got all excited and was determined to make me his personal protégé. He took me up to Candler School of Theology and introduced me around and we began the application process. I got cold feet, however, for reasons I am not even sure of, and never did follow through. Instead, I devoted myself to teaching and coaching and telling myself that I could serve the Lord in a lot of ways other than preaching.

In some ways, I have, but as I lay in bed at Salem that week, thinking about all that had gone on in my life, I knew that if I were ever going to know that perfect peace that would only come from being in totally alignment with God's plan for my life, we had to get this preacher thing settled once and for all.

As I lay in my bed, trying to get to sleep, I willed my mind to drift back to the idyllic days of my childhood, growing up in Porterdale without a care in the world. As I have related before, we could be out the door in Porterdale as soon as the sun came up and didn't have to be back in the house until the streetlight came on or our mothers called us for supper.

A lot of times, though, if I was having a real good time doing whatever it was I was doing, I wouldn't even answer her call. I would pretend I had not heard her. It never worked out very well. First she would just call "Darrell!" If I didn't respond right away she would throw that middle name in there, "Darrell Lee! Darrell Lee! You'd better get in this house!"

I am convinced that the only reason Southerners have two names is for when they get in trouble with their mamas. If she ever got to "Darrell Lee Huckaby!" I knew there was going to be a butt-whipping involved.

She would always say the same thing to me. "You heard me calling you! Why didn't you answer me?"

The answer I would invariably mumble in reply was never sufficient and she would send me to cut a switch.

That night I lay in my bed at Salem, realizing that although I was better and thought I was going to be OK, I knew there was the possibility of my dying relatively soon, but I knew the possibility of dying eventually was an absolute certainty. I promised God that very night that if He would still have me, I would do everything I could to preach the gospel of Jesus Christ every chance I got.

It was one thing to have Tommie Huckaby send me to cut a switch. I didn't want to face Jesus and hear Him say, "Darrell Lee; didn't you hear me calling you?" I think Jesus uses a winnowing rod, which is probably a lot worse than a switch.

The very next night, at the evening service, I looked across the big open-air tabernacle and saw a contingent of folks from Julia A. Porter walking up to take their seats in the pews. We still had a few minutes before the music was to begin, so I got up and walked around to greet them. Walter and Ann Pope, two lifelong friends, got me off to the side and said they had something to ask me. They wanted to know if I would deliver the Homecoming service in October at my childhood church.

I couldn't have been more honored if Sam Ramsey had invited me to be the preacher of the week at Salem. Well, not too much more honored.

That was most assuredly a God-incidence and a message from above that I was making the right choice. I had no idea, however, how to pursue the ministry at my advanced age. I was in a good place to find out, though. Over the next few days, I spent a lot of time discussing the calling I knew I had and was finally ready to answer that call with two of the best people I know, Alice Rogers and Bishop Bubba. Dr. Alice Rogers is an ordained elder in the United Methodist Church and is currently on the faculty at the Candler School of Theology. Bubba—or Reverend Hugh as I suppose he prefers to be called when he is anywhere except Salem—is also an ordained United Methodist elder and serves two churches in the Elberton-Athens District of the North Georgia Conference.

Both Alice and Hugh were eager to listen to what I had to say without trying to tell me what I needed to do. They laid out my options and urged me to pray about it. "There are many paths you can take," Alice counseled me, "and you need to just make sure you choose the one that allows you to do what you and God wants you to do, which is preach the word."

I assured her that my skill set didn't involve pastoring a church. I am not anywhere close to being organized enough to do that. I feel the call to evangelize, to preach Christ crucified and to help bring the light of Christ into a dark world that is growing darker, I fear, every day.

I left camp meeting that Friday night thankful that God had allowed me to get well enough to try and make things completely right with Him after all these years. I left camp meeting determined that I was going to use the time I had left to finally become a Methodist preacher.

There was one little sticking point, however. First I had to become a Methodist.

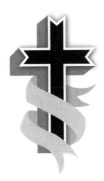

CHAPTER THIRTY FOUR

I was a Methodist for nine months before I was born. I have never really left the Methodist Church in spirit, but a few years ago we began attending Rockdale Baptist Church, where Lisa had been raised, primarily because their very strong youth program suited our needs at the time better than any other in the community. Plus, Lisa wanted a chance to worship with her family and lifelong friends. She had always gone to the church of my choice and I knew this was the right move at the time.

Rockdale Baptist was, indeed, the right choice for us at the time. It is filled with wonderful people, people who love us and our children and people who rejoiced when we announced that we were joining. I taught an adult Sunday school class for years and we made friends in that class that will remain our closest friends for the rest of our natural lives.

But I was determined to answer the call I had received from God as a teenager to become a Methodist minister, and as I had learned from Alice Rogers, the United Methodist church has many paths to help me reach my goal. Just as I knew that joining Rockdale Baptist had been the right thing to do for our family at the time, I knew now that re-joining the United Methodist Church was the right move at this time.

I made a lunch appointment with Conyers First UMC Senior Pastor, Reverend John Beyers. John and I had known each other for about five years and we had become good friends, once he forgave me for writing in one of my columns that he had the whitest legs I had ever seen. I had worshipped at First Methodist on many occasions over the five years John had served there, and he always appreciated my dropping by to "pay my respects to Mr. Wesley," as he put it.

He knew I was more comfortable worshipping in the Methodist tradition and let me know at every opportunity that he hoped one day to welcome me back into the United Methodist fold. He had invited me to speak at his church on a number of occasions and my attendance there had become more and more regular since I had been diagnosed with cancer.

We talked about my decision over Italian food—John chose the restaurant; I am not sure if there was any significance to the choice—and he was very, very supportive and pledged to do anything he could to help me understand the true nature of my calling, decide what path to pursue, and to help expedite the process.

He did remind me, quite gently, that I had to be a member of a United Methodist church to become a United Methodist preacher, be it a certified lay speaker, a licensed pastor of a small church, or a fully ordained elder.

I was prepared for that and assured him that Lisa and I were prepared to join at the first possible opportunity, which would be that Sunday. I was very relieved when John assured me that the following Sunday would be perfect. The first time Lisa and I joined a church together as husband and wife, we went to meet with the pastor and tell him that we wanted to come down front and join the church the following Sunday, We were told, "Next Sunday isn't really a good day to do that. How would three weeks from now work for you?"

Gracious! How can any Sunday not be a good Sunday to join the church?

John sent me to talk with Debbie Golden, who takes care of such matters at CFUMC and who happens to be the most organized person I have ever known, and everything was taken care of—everything except leaving the Baptist church.

I wanted to do that the right way and didn't want any misconceptions or bruised feelings, so I made an appointment with Rockdale's

Senior Pastor, Billy Moss, to explain to him what was going on and why we were leaving the church. He was delighted. In fact, relieved might have been a better word, and he asked me to address the congregation the following Sunday to share my good news.

I was happy to do so, but stood at the pulpit with mixed emotions. I stared out at the congregation and saw the faces of Benny and Bitzi, Lisa's parents, and Fred and Colleen Gordon, who were like her parents—in fact Colleen claims me as one of her own, and I am happy to claim her. Then there was Marie Stewart, who hasn't let a month go by without sending me a card or prayer-gram, and Martha and Bob Mann, who are like another set of parents to me—not to mention all the friends in our Sunday school class. You can call it a small group if you want to. I still call it a Sunday school class.

Somehow I got through my testimony and explained why I had decided, at that late date, to answer the call to preach. To my amazement, my remarks were met not with polite applause as I had expected, but a genuine heart-felt standing ovation. And I don't think it was because they were happy to get rid of me, either. I am pretty sure it was as sincere as it could have possibly been.

It was really quite an unusual day. We left one church at 9:30 and joined another at noon. I was reminded of a great scene from one of the funniest movies ever produced, O Brother Where Art Thou? Everett, the character played by George Clooney, was explaining to Baby Face Nelson that Pete and Delmar had recently been baptized and that Tommy had just sold his soul to the devil. "I'm the only one," boasted Everett, "that remains unaffiliated, in a manner of speaking."

For a couple of hours, Lisa and I were unaffiliated, in a manner of speaking. Not really, though. We have both known our whole life whose we are.

I still had a lot of speaking engagements lined up. The Homecoming service at Ray's United Methodist, Jerry Varnado's church, was amazing. People just kept coming in and kept coming in. The start of the service was held up about fifteen minutes while we got all the people in the door and found them a place to sit or stand. I was so proud to be able to stand in that pulpit and tell those good people how something positive and good had come out of something as bad as cancer. I am not saying, mind you, that God gave me cancer to get my attention. I can't imagine that a loving God would do something like that. I am saying, however, that something good came out of my having cancer—and God is and will continue to be glorified as the prayers still being lifted up by the thousands continue to be answered in a positive way.

On the first day of August, I spoke at a senior citizen's luncheon at Zion Baptist Church near Conyers. Lisa's uncle, Larry Potts, and her aunt, Betty, have been faithful members of Zion for a long, long time. Larry had been fighting leukemia for a long time and hadn't been able to get to church in months. He was the first person I saw when I walked into the fellowship hall.

I had never been happier to see someone in my life. He was dressed up and had a smile on his face and everybody in the hall was thrilled to see him. I was so honored that he had come to hear me talk, as bad off as he was. After seeing all the women of the church flocking to hug his neck, I told him that I thought he had come to see all the ladies instead of me.

Larry died eight days later.

Now here I am, back in the swing of things, teaching the history of this great nation to young people—every other day, instead of five days a week—writing my columns, speaking whenever and wherever I can, and listening for the still sweet voice of God to guide me in the exact direction He would have me go.

I still have a few balls up in the air. A recent bone scan has revealed that, while my cancer is still contained in the same area of my bones as it had been, I am suffering bone degeneration in my shoulders and hips, probably from arthritis, according to Dr. Pagliaro. Funny. I never thought I'd be happy to hear that I had arthritis. I made a visit to M.D. Anderson as I was preparing to put this book to bed, as they say in the trade, and was delighted to learn that my PSA remains undetectable, six months after beginning treatment.

I was not quite so delighted that the Lupron injections still hurt like a son of a gun.

I am still fatigued and in a lot of pain some days and I still have a lot of mysterious pain in my stomach and chest that none of my doctors seem able to diagnose or treat. Maybe that's just the thorn in my side that St. Paul spoke of so eloquently. Or maybe it's just the after-effects of getting knocked off a ladder by a tree limb, like Gary said to begin with.

But I am here.

In the last two years I have had three major surgeries, forty external beam radiation treatments, four nuclear body scans, several tests that I can't recall, had my blood tested dozens of times and have seen twenty-three different doctors. I still have Stage 4 metastatic prostate disease and there is still no cure. But I am still standing. As former Lester Maddox used to tell me every Saturday, "I woke up this morning. A lot of folks didn't."

"Yea, though I walk through the valley of the shadow of death I will fear no evil." King David wrote that—what?—3,500 years ago. I still pray it, and believe it, several times a day.

Over the past two years I have received thousands of cards, letters and notes, more than a million Facebook likes of my positive posts, more messages and posts than I could possibly count, and more acts of love and kindness from a legion of friends and followers, individuals and groups, than I could begin to acknowledge. And more prayers than anyone could possibly count, except for the one to whom they were delivered. He knows about each and every one of them. I guarantee it.

"My cup runneth over. Surely goodness and mercy shall follow me all the days of my life."

As for becoming a United Methodist minister—there are a lot of questions that have to be answered before I head down that path. I am in contact with the folks at Candler, although a lot of my minister friends are advising me that I have so much to say and do and that the seminary requires so many years of time that I might want to take a shorter path. I have already completed the United Methodist Church's Basic Lay Speaker's class. The one I took happened to be at Ray's United Methodist—Jerry Varnado's church, where I preached the Homecoming message in July. Coincidence? I think not.

By the time you read this, whomever you may be, I should have completed the advanced class and be a fully Certified Lay Speaker.

Give me a call, no matter your denomination or affiliation. I have a powerful message to bring—a message of salvation through the grace of a risen Savior. It's been more than 2,000 years and folks are still talking about it. And to think, He died for a sinner like me—and you.

"How then shall they call on Him in whom they have not believed? And how shall they believe in Him of whom they have not heard? And how shall they hear without a preacher?" Paul wrote that in Romans 10:14. I am ready to live it and know God will let me in His own time and in His own way.

Here am I, Lord. Send me.

I don't know how this story is going to turn out, but I know it is going to have a happy ending.

Thank you for joining me on my journey.

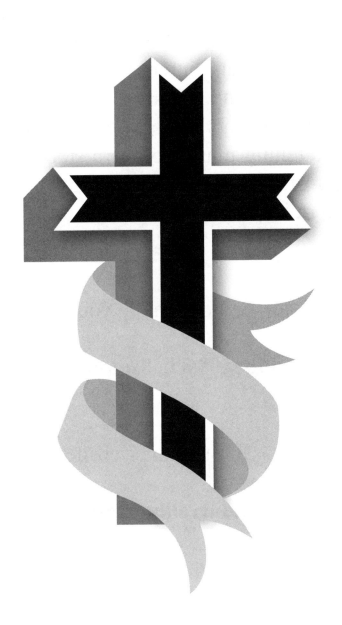

Darrell Huckaby is a Certified Lay Speaker in the United Methodist Church and speaks and preaches at churches of all denominations. He also entertains at civic functions and corporate events across the nation—and enjoys telling funny Southern stories to any group of people who enjoy laughter and a touch of inspiration.

Contact him to speak to your group at

dhuck08@bellsouth.net

or through his website.

www.darrellhuckaby.net

Other great books by Darrell Huckaby
available at

www.darrellhuckaby.net

Need Two
the funniest book ever written about college football

Dinner on the Grounds
the ultimate church cookbook

Grits is Groceries
and other facts of Southern life

Southern is as Southern Does
a linthead looks at life

Need Four
the further adventures of Whit and Andrew

What the Huck!
The Wit and Wisdom of the Last Southerner

A Southerner Looks at **All Fifty** *States*

Second Helpings
the Southern Eatin' Cookbook